Careers in Focus

Alternative Health Care

Ferguson Publishing Company
Chicago, Illinois

Copyright © 1999 Ferguson Publishing Company
ISBN 0-89434-283-5

Library of Congress Cataloging-in-Publication Data

Careers in Focus.   Alternative Health Care
     p.   cm.
  ISBN 0-89434-246-0
  1. Alternative medicine—Vocational guidance. I. Title: Alternative health
care.
R733.C365   1999   99-34039
610—dc21   CIP

Printed in the United States of America

Cover photo courtesy FPG

Published and distributed by
Ferguson Publishing Company
200 West Jackson Boulevard, 7th Floor
Chicago, Illinois 60606
312-692-1000

W-8

Table of Contents

Introduction

The field of alternative health care is not actually an established industry with a defined structure and branches. Alternative health care is a diverse collection of approaches to wellness, health care, and medicine. Its modalities can roughly be grouped into three categories: ancient traditional medical systems, more recent complete medical systems, and individual therapies.

Traditional medical systems, such as Ayurveda (traditional Indian medicine) and Oriental medicine, have been developed and practiced over hundreds of years in the cultures of their origin. These traditional systems are based upon complete philosophies regarding the origins and nature of life, human beings, wellness, and medicine. To successfully learn and practice such systems, you must be open to understanding and integrating a different value system and worldview into your approach to life and the practice of health care and medicine.

A number of alternative approaches are of more recent origin but also represent complete health care systems. Learning such health care systems, including homeopathy and chiropractic, does not require the acquisition of a different philosophy, but many of them require an educational process that is as demanding as the study of conventional medicine.

Other alternative health care approaches focus on a particular type of therapy. Examples of this group are aromatherapy and massage therapy. These therapies are not complete systems of health care. Many of them can be incorporated into the practices of other health practitioners. The therapies generally require less intensive education, but they provide very meaningful opportunities to help people improve their lives.

With its emphasis on wellness, cooperation, and the whole person, the field of alternative health care has brought a new sense of enthusiasm, innovation, and hope to patients, to health care, and to the medical profession. The rapid changes that have occurred in health care and medicine in recent years seem to have a life and momentum of their own. Where will all of this change and enthusiasm lead?

In late 1998, the U.S. government gave additional recognition to the field of alternative health care. It elevated the Office of Alternative Medicine (OAM) to the status of a center—the National Center for Complementary and Alternative Medicine (NCCAM). It also dramatically increased NCCAM's budget from $20 million in 1998 to $50 million for fiscal year 1999. The center will focus on conducting clinical trials in a variety of alternative approaches. These trials may provide scientific data that will help legitimize alternative approaches in the eyes of conventional practitioners and thus help pave the way toward more cooperation between alternative and conventional practitioners.

With its hope, excitement, and change, alternative health care is the most rapidly growing segment of the field of health care in general. Significant recent events indicate that the alternative health care explosion will continue well into the 21st century.

Each article in this book discusses a particular alternative health care occupation in detail. The information comes from Ferguson's *Encyclopedia of Careers and Vocational Guidance.* The History section describes the history of the particular job as it relates to the overall development of its industry or field. The Job describes the primary and secondary duties of the job. Requirements discusses high school and postsecondary education and training requirements, any certification or licensing necessary, and any other personal requirements for success in the job. Exploring offers suggestions on how to gain some experience in or knowledge of the particular job before making a firm educational and financial commitment. The focus is on what can be done while still in high school (or in the early years of college) to gain a better understanding of the job. The Employers section gives an overview of typical places of employment for the job. Starting Out discusses the best ways to land that first job, be it through the college placement office, newspaper ads, or personal contact. The Advancement section describes what kind of career path to expect from the job and how to get there. Earnings lists salary ranges and describes the typical fringe benefits. The Work Environment section describes the typical surroundings and conditions of employment—whether indoors or outdoors, noisy or quiet, social or independent, and so on. Also discussed are typical hours worked, any seasonal fluctuations, and the stresses and strains of the job. The Outlook section summarizes the job in terms of the general economy and industry projections. For the most part, Outlook information is obtained from the Bureau of Labor Statistics and is supplemented by information taken from professional associations.

Job growth terms follow those used in the *Occupational Outlook Handbook:* Growth described as "much faster than the average" means an increase of 36 percent or more. Growth described as "faster than the average" means an increase of 21 to 35 percent. Growth described as "about as fast as the average" means an increase of 10 to 20 percent. Growth described as "little change or more slowly than the average" means an increase of 0 to 9 percent. "Decline" means a decrease of 1 percent or more.

Each article ends with For More Information, which lists organizations that can provide career information on training, education, internships, scholarships, and job placement.

Acupuncturists

School Subjects
| Biology
| Business
| Psychology

Personal Skills
| Helping/teaching
| Technical/scientific

Work Environment
| Primarily indoors
| Primarily one location

Minimum Education Level
| Associate's degree

Salary Range
| $13,000 to $40,000 to $100,000

Certification or Licensing
| Required by certain states

Outlook
| Much faster than the average

Overview

Acupuncturists are health care professionals who practice the ancient Oriental healing art of acupuncture. Acupuncture is a complete medical system that encourages the body to improve functioning and promote natural healing. It has been practiced in China for thousands of years to maintain health, prevent disease, treat illness, and alleviate pain. It has been proven to be effective in the treatment of emotional and psychological problems as well as physical ailments.

In 1997, there were approximately 10,000 professional acupuncturists in the United States. In addition, about 3,000 medical doctors have been trained in acupuncture. Acupuncture is one of the fastest growing health care professions. Most acupuncturists work in private practice, although an increasing number work in clinics and hospitals.

History

Acupuncture has been practiced for thousands of years. It is one of the ancient Chinese healing arts. The Chinese believe that acupuncture began during the Stone Age. They think that early people used sharp stone tools to puncture and drain boils. As time passed, primitive needles made of stone or pottery replaced the earlier tools. They, in turn, were replaced by metal needles, which evolved into the very thin needles acupuncturists use today.

Early metal needles had nine different shapes, and they were used for a variety of purposes. However, there were no specific points on the body where they were applied. Through centuries of experience and observation, the Chinese learned that the use of the needles on very specific points on the skin was effective in treating particular ailments. They later grouped specific acupuncture points into a system of channels, or *meridians*. Acupuncturists think that these channels run over and through the body, much like rivers and streams run over and through the earth. They teach that the body has a type of vital energy, called *qi* or *chi* (both are pronounced "chee"), and that this energy flows through the body. The acupuncture points along the channels are thought to influence the flow of the vital energy.

Acupuncture developed virtually uninterrupted over thousands of years until the Portuguese landed in China in 1504. Once China was opened to the rest of the world, Western medical concepts gradually began to influence the practice of medicine there. Over centuries, the practice of acupuncture declined, and in 1929, it was outlawed in China. Even so, it remained a part of the folk medicine. When the Communist Party came to power in 1949, there were almost no medical services. The communists encouraged the use of traditional Chinese remedies, and acupuncture again began to grow.

Just as Western medicine filtered into China, the concept of acupuncture gradually travelled back to the West. It was probably known and used in Europe as early as the 17th century. The first recorded use was in 1810 at the Paris Medical School where Dr. Berlioz used it to treat abdominal pain. Acupuncture was also used in England in the early 1800s. Ear acupuncture, one of the newer forms of acupuncture, was largely developed outside of China. In the early 1950s, Dr. Paul Nogier of France developed the detailed map of the ear that most acupuncturists now use.

After President Nixon visited China in 1972, public awareness and use of acupuncture began to grow in North America. Today acupuncture is increasingly used in Europe, North America, and Russia. Over one-third of the world's population relies on acupuncture and Oriental medicine practitioners for prevention and treatment of disease, as well as for the enhancement of health. In the West, acupuncture is most well-known for pain relief, but a growing body of research shows that it is effective in health maintenance as well as the treatment of many diseases. In 1979, the World Health Organization (WHO), the medical branch of the United Nations, issued a list of more than 40 diseases and other health conditions that acupuncture helped alleviate.

During the last decade of the 20th century, major developments in the perception of health care in this country and throughout the world have brought acupuncture and Oriental medicine to the forefront of health care. In 1996, the Food and Drug Administration (FDA) reclassified acupuncture needles from "investigational" to "safe and effective" medical devices. This opened the door for acupuncture to be covered for insurance reimbursement. The 1997 report sponsored by the National Institutes of Health (NIH) concluded that acupuncture should be integrated into standard medical practice and included in Medicare. These milestones have paved the way toward greater acceptance of acupuncture by the medical community and by the American public.

The Job

Acupuncture is the best-known component of a larger system of medicine, known as Oriental medicine. Oriental medicine encompasses a variety of healing modalities, including acupuncture, Chinese herbology, bodywork, dietary therapy, and exercise. An Oriental medicine practitioner may practice them all or specialize in only one or two.

Acupuncturists treat symptoms and disorders by inserting very thin needles into precise acupuncture points on the skin. They believe that the body's qi flows along specific channels in the body. Each channel is related to a particular physiological system and internal organ. Disease, pain, and other physical and emotional conditions result when the body's qi is unbalanced, or when the flow of qi along the channels is blocked or disrupted. Acupuncturists stimulate the acupuncture points to balance the circulation of energy. This influences the health of the whole person. The purpose of acupuncture and other forms of traditional Oriental medicine is to restore and maintain balance in the body's qi.

Those who practice acupuncture believe that when qi is balanced, the person is healthy. Acupuncture has been used for centuries to maintain health by maintaining the balance of qi. It is also used to relieve a wide range of common ailments, including asthma, high blood pressure, headache, and back pain. A recent important use of acupuncture is for treatment of substance abuse withdrawal. Some areas of medicine that use acupuncture include internal medicine, oncology, obstetrics and gynecology, pediatrics, urology, geriatrics, sports medicine, immunology, infectious diseases, and psychiatric disorders. In the United States, acupuncture is perhaps most frequently used for relief of pain.

Like many other health care professionals, acupuncturists take an initial health history when they receive a new patient. They need to know about the patient's past and present problems. They listen carefully and sensitively, and they incorporate the patient history into their plan of treatment.

Next, acupuncturists give a physical examination. During the examination, they try to determine if a patient's qi is unbalanced. If it is, they look for the location of the imbalance. They test the quality of the pulses in both of the patient's wrists. They examine the shape and color of the tongue, skin color, body language, and tone of voice. They also check the feel of diagnostic areas of the body, such as the back and the abdomen. Acupuncturists may test for weaknesses in the muscles or along the meridians.

Once acupuncturists identify the source of the qi imbalance, they choose the type of needle to be used. There are nine types of acupuncture needles, ranging from just over an inch to as long as seven inches. Each type of needle is used to treat certain conditions. Most acupuncturists in the United States and other Western countries use only three types of needles that range from one to three inches in length. After selecting the type of needle, acupuncturists determine where the needles will be inserted on the patient's body. There are thousands of possible insertion points on the body. Four to twelve needles are typically used in a treatment.

Acupuncture needles are flexible. They are about the diameter of a human hair—much thinner than injection-type needles. They are inserted to a depth of up to an inch. Insertion of the needles is generally painless, although sensitive individuals may feel fleeting discomfort. During treatment, acupuncturists may stimulate the needles to increase the effect. Stimulation is done by twirling the needles or by applying heat or a low electrical current to them.

The first visit usually lasts an hour or more because the history and physical require extra time. Follow-up visits are usually shorter—perhaps 15 to 45 minutes, although treatments sometimes last an hour or longer. Occasionally only one treatment is required. Other times, the patient may have to return for several sessions. The number needed varies according to the individual. The number of treatments needed varies according to the situation.

If acupuncturists incorporate other modalities of Oriental medicine into their practices, they may supplement the acupuncture with the other treatments. They might include herbal therapy, massage, exercise, or nutritional counseling.

In addition to treating patients, acupuncturists have a number of other duties. Most are self-employed, so they have to do their own paperwork. They write reports on their patients' treatments and progress. They bill insurance companies to make sure they get paid. They also have to market their services in order to build their clientele. It is important for them to maintain contacts with other professionals in the medical community; other professionals may be good sources of referrals. Acupuncturists must also keep up with developments and changes in their profession through continuing education.

Requirements

High School

If you are interested in a career in acupuncture, you need to take courses that will give you an understanding of the human body. Courses in biology, physiology, and psychology will help you gain an understanding of the body and insight into the mind. You also need to take courses that prepare you for college entrance. Good communication skills are important in all professions. English, speech, drama, and debate can help you develop your communication skills.

You are likely to be self-employed if you become an acupuncturist, so math, business, and computer courses will also be helpful. A good, well-rounded education will help prepare you for any career you might choose.

Postsecondary Training

More than 60 schools in the United States offer courses in acupuncture. The national professional associations listed at the end of this chapter can supply you with the names, addresses, and descriptions of the programs. Most offer master's level programs. To be admitted into a master's level program in acupuncture, virtually every school requires a minimum of two years of undergraduate study. Others require a bachelor's degree in a related field, such as science, nursing, or premed. Most acupuncture programs provide a thorough education in Western sciences, acupuncture techniques, and all aspects of traditional Oriental medicine.

Choosing a school for acupuncture can be complex. The national professional associations have information to assist you with this. One important decision is where you might like to live and practice. Eligibility requirements vary from state to state, so it is important to be sure the school you choose will prepare you to practice in the state in which you wish to live. In some states, only physicians can be licensed to practice acupuncture. In other states, there are no requirements for practicing acupuncture.

Another consideration in making a school choice is the tradition of acupuncture you want to study. There are a number of different types of acupuncture. You will need to find a school that offers the type that interests you. If you will need financial assistance, it is important to choose a college that is accredited by the Accreditation Commission for Acupuncture and Oriental Medicine (ACAOM). The U.S. Department of Education recognizes programs accredited by the ACAOM. If you are enrolled in an accredited program, you may be eligible for federal student loans.

Certification or Licensing

For acupuncture, certification indicates that an individual meets the standards established by a nationally recognized commission. Licensing is a requirement established by a state's governmental body that grants individuals the right to practice within that state. Licensing requirements vary widely around the country and are changing rapidly. More than 30 states license acupuncturists.

Licensing is achieved by meeting educational and exam requirements. The National Certification Commission for Acupuncture and Oriental Medicine (NCCAOM) certifies acupuncturists and promotes nationally recognized standards for acupuncture and Oriental medicine. Virtually every state uses NCCAOM's test for licensing purposes. If you graduate from a school in the United States, you must complete a three-year ACAOM-accredited or master's level program in order to take NCCAOM's exam. If you graduate from a school outside the United States, the program must be judged to be equivalent. The national professional organizations are great sources for the most up-to-date information about certification and licensing issues.

The nationwide trend is toward more education and stricter certification and licensing requirements. The profession is developing the Doctor of Oriental Medicine designation, which should be available in the near future.

Other Requirements

Like other health care practitioners, acupuncturists frequently work with people who are in pain and who have been ill for a long time. Patients often come to acupuncturists after other medical treatments have failed. They may be especially pessimistic about finding relief or cures. Acupuncturists need to be good listeners, patient, and compassionate. Acupuncturists also need to have sensitive hands.

Claudette Baker, Lic. Ac. (licensed acupuncturist), has her office in Evanston, Illinois. She believes that people who become acupuncturists need to have a special perspective on health care. According to her, "Those who consider a career in acupuncture should be interested in medicine and in healing, but they should also be aware that this profession requires a change in their perception of medicine. Oriental medicine is a science of understanding energetics in the body, and it is a healing art. Students should only consider acupuncture if they have an aptitude for understanding and learning this approach to medicine."

Exploring

If a career in acupuncture interests you, there are many ways to learn more about it. You will find many books at the library. Studying Oriental history, thought, and philosophy will help you learn to understand Oriental medicine's approach to healing.

Health food stores sometimes have books on acupuncture, and they are good places to learn about other alternative/complementary health modalities. Ask the staff if they know acupuncturists in your area. Talk with people who have experienced acupuncture. Find out what it was like and how they felt about it. Make an appointment for a health consultation with an acupuncturist. Find out if this approach to medicine works for you, and if you would like to use it to help others.

Read about or take courses in yoga or t'ai qi (t'ai chi). These are ancient methods for achieving control of the mind and body, and the principles on which they are based are similar to those of acupuncture.

Learn about the national and state professional associations. Some of them offer student memberships. Many of them have excellent information online. Others have materials available for sale at reasonable prices.

Visit colleges of acupuncture. Sit in on classes. Talk to the students. Find out what it is like to be a student of acupuncture. Ask what they like and what they don't like.

Attend meetings of professional organizations. Get to know the people and the issues in the field. By networking with experienced acupuncturists, you can learn a lot and may even find a mentor.

Employers

Most acupuncturists operate private practices. Some form or join partnerships with other acupuncturists or with people skilled in other areas of Oriental medicine. Professionals and clinics in other areas of health care, such as chiropractors, osteopaths, and medical doctors, increasingly include acupuncturists among them.

As acupuncture is finding more acceptance, there are growing opportunities for acupuncturists in hospitals and university medical schools. A few acupuncturists are engaged in medical research. They conduct studies on the effectiveness of acupuncture in treating various health conditions. There is a growing emphasis on research in acupuncture, and this area is likely to employ greater numbers in the future. A small number of acupuncturists work for government agencies, such as the National Institutes of Health.

Starting Out

To get started as an acupuncturist, one of the most important elements is being sure that you have the proper certification and licensing for your geographical area. This bears repeating, since the requirements for the profession, for each state, and for the nation are changing so rapidly.

The placement office of your school may be able to help you find job opportunities. When starting out, some acupuncturists find jobs in clinics with doctors or chiropractors or in wellness centers. This gives them a chance to start practicing without having to equip an office. Some begin working with a more experienced acupuncturist and then later go into private practice. Acupuncturists frequently work in private practice. When starting a new practice, they often have full-time jobs and begin their practices part time.

Networking with professionals in local and national organizations is a good way to learn about job opportunities.

Advancement

Acupuncturists advance in their careers by establishing their own practices and by building large bases of patients. Some start their own clinics. Because acupuncturists receive referrals from physicians and other health care practitioners, relationships with other members of the medical community can be very helpful in building a patient base.

Acupuncturists may eventually wish to teach acupuncture at a school of Oriental medicine. After much experience, an acupuncturist may achieve a supervisory or directorship position in a school. The growing acceptance of acupuncture by the American public and the medical community will lead to an increasing need for research. Acupuncturists can build rewarding careers participating in this effort.

Earnings

Barbara Mitchell, Executive Director of the National Acupuncture and Oriental Medicine Alliance, stated that an informal 1998 survey of their members found that starting pay for a private practitioner may be $13,000 to $20,000 until the practice grows. As with any other form of self-employment, income is directly related to the number of hours you work and the rate you can charge. Rates increase with experience.

An average income for a full-time acupuncturist would be $30,000 to $40,000. Physicians who practice acupuncture as part of their medical practices have incomes well over $100,000. A very experienced acupuncturist with a well-established medical practice can sometimes net $200,000 or more.

Work Environment

Acupuncturists usually work indoors in clean, quiet, comfortable offices. Since most are in solo practice, they can choose their surroundings. Private practitioners set their own hours, but many work some evenings and weekends to accommodate their patients' schedules. They usually work without supervision and must have a lot of self-discipline. Like other self-employed individuals, acupuncturists must provide their own insurance, vacation, and retirement benefits.

For acupuncturists who work in clinics, hospitals, and universities, the surroundings vary. They may work in large hospitals or small colleges. However, wherever they work, acupuncturists need clean, quiet offices. In these larger settings, acupuncturists need to be able to work well in a team environment. They may also need to be able to work well under supervision. Those who are employed in these organizations usually receive salaries and benefits. They may have to follow hours set by the employer.

Outlook

Acupuncture is growing very rapidly as a profession due to increasing public awareness and acceptance. The recent advances in research, changes in government policy, and interest from the mainstream medical community are strong indicators that the field will continue to expand. As insurance, HMO (health maintenance organization), and other third-party reimbursements increase, acupuncture is expected to grow even more rapidly. In 1997, the World Health Organization (the medical branch of the United Nations) estimated that there were over 10,000 acupuncture specialists in the United States. The number of certified and licensed acupuncturists is expected to increase as additional states establish legal guidelines for acupuncturists.

The number of people who receive acupuncture treatments is growing annually. One of the areas of greatest growth is in the treatment of addictions. The United States has provided more than one million dollars for research programs to investigate acupuncture's effect on cocaine addiction and alcoholism. Many hospitals and prisons now use acupuncture in their substance abuse programs. Besides the treatment of addictions, other areas of increase in acupuncture include the treatment of chronic pain, bronchial asthma, and premenstrual syndrome.

Despite these factors favoring job growth, much education and research still need to be done to integrate this system of natural healing into the conventional American health care system.

For More Information

For general information, comprehensive information on the legal status of acupuncture and Oriental medicine in individual states, a list of schools, and a Web site with good links, contact:

American Association of Oriental Medicine
433 Front Street
Catasauqua, PA 18032
Tel: 610-266-1433
Web: http://www.aaom.org

For a particularly active Web site with an online journal and updates on education and California legislation, visit:

California Association of Acupuncture & Oriental Medicine
1231 State Street, Suite 208A
Santa Barbara, CA 92101
Tel: 800-477-4564
Web: http//www.caaom.org

For information on academic guidelines, contact:

Council of Colleges of Acupuncture and Oriental Medicine
1010 Wayne Avenue, Suite 1270
Silver Spring, MD 20910
Tel: 301-608-9175
Web: http//www.ccaom.org

For information for potential students, general information about acupuncture and Oriental medicine, and thorough information about national organizations, changes in legislation, and state standards, contact:

National Acupuncture and Oriental Medicine Alliance
14637 Starr Road SE
Olalla, WA 98359
Tel: 253-851-6896
Web: http://www.acuall.org

Aromatherapists

Biology Chemistry English	School Subjects
Helping/teaching Technical/scientific	Personal Skills
Primarily indoors Primarily one location	Work Environment
Some postsecondary training	Minimum Education Level
$13,000 to $30,000 to $70,000+	Salary Range
None available	Certification or Licensing
Faster than the average	Outlook

Overview

Aromatherapists are health care specialists who use a deep understanding of the principles of aromatherapy to help their clients live healthier, more satisfying lives. Aromatherapy is the science and art of using essential plant oils to promote health. Essential oils are highly concentrated substances that give plants their fragrance. These substances are extracted from various parts of aromatic plants—roots, woods, seeds, fruits, leaves, and flowers, among others. Only about 5 percent of all types of plants are used for their essential oils.

Since the early 20th century, the professions of cosmetology, medicine, and psychology have rediscovered the healing powers of essential oils that were known to earlier civilizations. Scientific studies show that inhaling the fragrance of certain essential oils has physiological and psychological effects on the brain. Aromatherapists study the oils and their effects on individuals. They use this knowledge to help improve their clients' quality of life.

Most aromatherapists are licensed in other areas of health care or body care. They study and practice aromatherapy as a healing modality that is supplementary to the profession in which they are licensed. Among these licensed professionals are beauticians, chiropractors, cosmeticians, massage therapists, medical doctors, naturopathic doctors, nurse practitioners, and nurses. A few individuals who specialize in aromatherapy work as chemists, educators, or authors. A very few grow plants for the distillation of essential oils, become consultants, or start their own lines of aromatherapy products.

History

In the spas of ancient Rome, oils were used in public baths and were applied during massages. The knowledge of oils went along with the spread of Roman culture. Europeans used oils during medieval times to fight disease. During the Middle Ages, the appearance of chemistry and the improvement of distillation helped simplify the process of extracting essential oils from plants. This opened the door to oil trading, which spread the new practices to more people and places.

Until the 19th century, when science began to introduce other medicines, Europeans used essential oils both as perfumes and for medicinal purposes. With the growth of newer medical practices, doctors began to choose modern medicine over the tradition of oils. It was not until the 20th century that several individuals "rediscovered" the healing power of essential oils. Once again the use of oils was integrated into Western culture.

In 1928, the French perfumer and chemist, René-Maurice Gattefossé, experienced the healing power of essential oils. When he severely burned his hand, he stuck it into the nearest liquid, which happened to be lavender oil. He was surprised how quickly the hand healed. His experience caused him to become interested in the therapeutic use of essential oils. It was Gattefossé who coined the term *aromatherapy*.

Dr. Jean Valnet, a French physician, was the first to reintegrate essential oils into Western medical practice. Dr. Valnet served as an army surgeon during World War II. Inspired by the work of Gattefossé, he used essential oils to treat the soldiers' burns and wounds. He also successfully treated psychiatric problems with fragrances. Marguerite Maury, an Austrian biochemist, was also influenced by the work of Gattefossé. She integrated the use of essential oils into cosmetics.

In 1977, Robert Tisserand, an expert in aromatherapy, wrote *The Art of Aromatherapy*. Tisserand was strongly influenced by the work of both Gattefossé and Valnet. His book caught the interest of the American public and made a major contribution to the growth of aromatherapy in this country.

The Western world has rediscovered the uses of essential oils and fragrances through the work of people like Valnet, Maury, and Tisserand. The world is reawakening to the healing and life-enhancing capabilities of aromatherapy.

The Job

Whether aromatherapists work primarily as beauticians, chiropractors, massage therapists, or doctors, they must possess a strong working knowledge of aromatherapy as a science and an art. They need to understand the components and healing benefits of many essential oils. The quality of essential oils varies greatly depending on the plant, where it is grown, the conditions under which it is grown, and other factors. As a result, aromatherapists must be very careful about choosing the sources from which their oils come. Pure, high quality, therapeutic grade oils are essential to good aromatherapy. Aromatherapists must even know the differences between the oils of different species of the same plant. Essential oils are very powerful because of their high concentration. It may take well over 100 pounds of plant material to produce just one pound of essential oil.

Because of the powerful concentration of essential oils, aromatherapists use great care in diluting them and in adding them to carriers. Carriers are most often high quality vegetable oils, such as almond, olive, or sesame. Unlike essential oils, carrier oils are fixed, rather than volatile. A small amount of an essential oil is blended into the carrier oil, which "carries" it across the body. Aromatherapists are especially careful when the oils are to be applied to a client's skin or put into a bath. In addition, aromatherapists must know how different essential oils work together because they combine oils to achieve certain results.

Aromatherapists need to know much more than what oils to use. They use the essential oils in three types of aromatherapy: cosmetic, massage, and olfactory. Aromatherapists have to know the differences among the types of therapy. They must decide which type or combination of types to use in a particular situation, and they must be skilled in each type.

Aromatherapists must know how the body, mind, and emotions work together. For example, a client who complains of muscle tension may need physical relief. A massage with relaxing oils that the skin soaks in will relax the client. However, aromatherapists are able to take this treatment a step further. They consider the underlying causes of the condition. Why is the client feeling tense? Is it stress? Anxiety? Strong emotion? Massage therapists who are trained in aromatherapy may inquire about the client's life in order to pinpoint the source of the tension. Once the source is identified, aromatherapists utilize specific oils to produce a certain emotional effect in the client. When the scents of these oils are inhaled, they create a response within the entire body. The oils may be added to a bath or a compress that is applied to the body. A compress is a towel soaked in water that has a bit of an essential oil added to it. An aroma may take the client back to happier times, as a reminder of warmth, comfort, and contentment.

An esthetician's client may have skin problems due to stress. The esthetician may use certain essential oils to help both the skin condition on the surface and the underlying emotional source of the problem. This might be accomplished through olfactory aromatherapy—the inhalation of the oil vapors.

In a hospital, nursing home, or hospice setting, an aromatherapist might choose essential oils that help relieve stress. In England, hospital nursing staffs utilize essential oil massage. This type of therapy has been shown to relieve pain and induce sleep. Essential oil massage has proven effective in relieving the stress that patients experience with general illness, surgery, terminal cancer, and AIDS. Aromatherapists emphasize that these treatments are supplementary and enhancing to medical care—they do not replace medical treatment.

No two clients' problems are the same, and neither are the remedies for those problems. Each client must be treated as an individual. During the first visit, aromatherapists usually take a careful client history. Aromatherapists must listen carefully for both those things their clients say and for those important things they don't say. Aromatherapists need to know if a client is taking any medicine or using any natural healing substances, such as herbs. They must understand the properties of the essential oils and how they might interact with any other treatment the client is using. Next, they use the information gathered from the client interview to determine the proper essential oils and the appropriate amounts to blend to serve the client's particular needs.

Aromatherapists are employed in a number of different work environments. Those connected to the beauty industry may work in salons, spas, or hotel resorts. They incorporate aromatherapy into facial care, body care, and hair care. In the health care field, many professionals are turning to alternative approaches to care, and some conventional medical practitioners are beginning to implement more holistic approaches. As a result, a growing number of aromatherapists work in the offices of other health care specialists where their aromatherapy treatments complement the other therapies used. Aromatherapists often give seminars, teach, or serve as consultants. Some who become experts on essential oils buy farms to grow plants for the oils, create their own lines of aromatherapy products, or sell essential oils to other aromatherapists.

Requirements

High School

Knowledge of the human body's systems is especially important to aromatherapy. Biology, anatomy, and physiology will help lay the foundation for a career in aromatherapy. Chemistry courses will familiarize you with laboratory procedures. Aromatherapists need to have an understanding of mixtures and the care involved in using powerful essential oils. Chemistry can help you gain the experience you need to handle delicate or volatile substances. It will also familiarize you with the properties of natural compounds.

Keep in mind that the majority of aromatherapists are self-employed. Math, business, and computer courses will help you develop the skills you need to be successful at running a business. Aromatherapists also need good communication and interpersonal skills to be sensitive to their clients. English, speech, and psychology classes can help you sharpen your ability to interact constructively with other people.

Eva-Marie Lind is the Dean of the Aromatherapy Department of the Australasian College of Herbal Studies in Lake Oswego, Oregon. She has worked in the field of aromatherapy for about 13 years. According to Lind, "Education is the key to good aromatherapy. There is so much to learn, and it takes real dedication to study."

Postsecondary Training

At this time, there are no educational requirements established for the field of aromatherapy. However, there are schools, seminars, and distance learning courses that offer training in aromatherapy. The programs range from short workshops to four-year college courses. Vocational schools, major universities, and naturopathic colleges are increasingly offering training in aromatherapy. Most courses include information about the human body and certain ailments. They also give extensive information on essential oils, how they work with one another, and how they enhance health. The Internet, professional magazines, and national associations are great sources of information and lists of programs and schools.

Since no educational standards have been established, you need to be particularly careful in your selection of programs. Call the schools or organizations that interest you. Ask how their programs are set up. For correspondence courses (or distance courses), ask if you will be able to talk to a teacher. How will you be evaluated? Are there tests? How are the tests taken and graded? Try to talk with current students. Ask how they are treated and what they learn. Ask what you receive when you graduate from the program. Will you receive help with job placement? Access to insurance programs? Other benefits?

Most aromatherapists are also professionals in other fields. Consider whether you would want to combine aromatherapy with a "base" profession, such as chiropractic, massage therapy, nursing, or some other field into which you might incorporate it. These base fields require additional education and certification as well as licensing. If you decide to add aromatherapy to another profession, learn the requirements for certification or licensing that apply to that profession. Adding aromatherapy to another profession requires a comprehensive understanding of both fields from a scientific standpoint.

Certification or Licensing

There are presently no certification or licensing requirements for aromatherapy in the United States. Aromatherapy is growing rapidly, and it is likely that these requirements will be established soon. Since aromatherapy is practiced by such a variety of professionals, developing standards is particularly complex. Geraldine Zelinsky, the 1998 public relations representative of the National Association for Holistic Aromatherapy (NAHA) says NAHA is working toward defining national accreditation and standards. Professionals throughout the industry are working toward developing standards. If you choose to study aromatherapy, you will need to keep up on these changes.

If you choose to combine aromatherapy with another profession, you must meet the national and local requirements for that field in addition to aromatherapy requirements.

Other Requirements

According to Eva-Marie Lind of the Australasian College of Herbal Studies, "Aromatherapy demands love and passion at its roots. You need to honor, respect, and celebrate the beauty of this field." You must also enjoy disseminating knowledge because clients often have many questions. More practically, it takes a good nose and a certain sensitivity to successfully treat clients through aromatherapy. It takes good listening skills and immense creativity to understand each client's personal issues and decide on the best means of administering a treatment. Which essential oils or combination of oils should you choose? Should you use a bath, a compress, a massage, or inhalation? What parts of the body are the best avenues for delivering the remedy?

Aromatherapists must be good self-teachers who are interested in continuing education. This is a relatively new field that is developing and changing rapidly. To stay competitive and successful, you need to keep up with the changing trends, products, and technologies that affect the field. Like most healing professions, aromatherapy is a lifelong education process for the practitioner.

Exploring

There are many ways to explore the field of aromatherapy to see if it is for you. For one, there are many books and specialized periodicals available on the subject. Get a glimpse of the types of knowledge you need for the field. Find out whether it is too scientific or not scientific enough. Look in your local library for books and magazines that show you what a typical student of aromatherapy might be learning.

Visit health food stores. The staff members of health food stores are often very helpful. Most have books, magazines, and newspapers about many kinds of alternative health care, including aromatherapy. Ask about essential oils, and ask for the names of aromatherapists in the area. Find out if there are garden clubs that you can join—particularly ones that specialize in herbs. Consider taking up cooking. This could give you practice in selecting herbs and seasonings and blending them to create different aromas and flavors.

Contact local and national professional organizations. Some offer student memberships or free seminars. Check out their Web sites. They have a lot of valuable information and good links to other alternative health care sites. Join online forums and discussion groups where you can communicate with professionals from all over the country and the world. Some distance learning courses are open to students of all ages. Check into them.

If you find you have a real interest in aromatherapy, another way to explore the field is to seek a mentor—a professional in the field who is willing to help you learn. Tell everyone you know that you are interested in aromatherapy. Someone is bound to have a connection with someone you could call for an informational interview. Perhaps you could spend a day "shadowing" an aromatherapist to see what the work is like. If you are unable to find an aromatherapy specialist, you could call spas and salons in search of professionals who use aromatherapy in their work. Perhaps some would be willing to speak to you about their day-to-day work. Make an appointment and experience an aromatherapy treatment. Taking it a step further, you could explore the possibility of getting a part-time job at an establishment that employs aromatherapists.

Employers

Most aromatherapists are self-employed. They run their own small business-es and build their own clientele. Some set up their own offices, but many build their businesses by working in the offices of other professionals and giving aromatherapy treatments as supplements to the treatments provided by the resident professionals. Many different kinds of employers are looking for skilled aromatherapists. In the cosmetic industry, beauticians, cosmeticians, and massage therapists employ aromatherapists to give treatments that complement their own. Spas, athletic clubs, resorts, and cruise ships may hire aromatherapists on a full-time basis. These types of employment may be temporary or seasonal.

In the health care industry, chiropractors, acupuncturists, and other alternative therapy practitioners and clinics may offer aromatherapy in addition to their basic services. Hospitals, nursing homes, hospice centers, and other medical establishments are beginning to recognize the physiological and psychological benefits of aromatherapy for their patients.

Starting Out

Because the practice of aromatherapy may be incorporated into numerous other professions, there are many ways to enter the field. How you enter depends on how you want to use aromatherapy. Is your interest in massage therapy, skin care, or hair care? Do you want to be a nurse, doctor, acupuncturist, or chiropractor? Are you interested in becoming an instructor or writer? Once you are certified in another area, you need to search for clinics, salons, spas, and other establishments that are looking for professionals who use aromatherapy in their treatments. School career services are also ways to find work. Classified ads in newspapers and trade magazines list positions in the related fields.

Networking can be an important source of job opportunities. Networking is simply getting to know others and exchanging ideas with them. Go to association meetings and conventions. Talk to people in the field. Job openings are often posted at such gatherings.

Advancement

Aromatherapists can advance to many different levels, depending on their goals, ambitions, aspirations, and willingness to work. Those who are self-employed can increase their clientele, open their own offices or even a salon. Those who are employed at a spa or salon could become a department director or the director of the entire spa or salon. They might start a private practice or open a spa or salon.

As their skills and knowledge grow, aromatherapists may be sought after to teach and train other aromatherapists in seminars or at schools that offer aromatherapy programs or courses. Others become consultants or write books and articles. A few start their own aromatherapy product lines of esthetic or therapeutic products. Some may become involved in growing the plants that are the sources of essential oils. Still others work in distilling, analyzing, or blending the oils.

This is such a new field growing so rapidly that the potential for advancement is enormous. The field has so many facets that the directions for growth are as great as your imagination and determination. Zelinsky of the National Association for Holistic Aromatherapists says, "If you are self-motivated, creative, and have a talent for any aspect of aromatherapy, the sky is the limit. It is what you make it."

Earnings

Since aromatherapists work in such a variety of settings, and aromatherapy is often a supplementary therapy added to other professional training, it is particularly difficult to make statements about average earnings in the field. Government agencies do not yet have wage statistics for the field. The national professional associations have not yet developed surveys of their members that give reliable information.

For those who are self-employed in any profession, earnings depend on the amount of time they work and the amount they charge per hour. Experienced professional aromatherapists estimate that hourly rates can range from $25 to $65 for beginning aromatherapists and instructors. Rates increase with experience to between $75 and $100 per hour. Based on those rates, a beginning aromatherapist who charged $25 an hour and averaged 10 appointments per week would earn around $13,000. Established aromatherapists who have a solid client base report earning $25,000 to $45,000.

The hourly rate you can charge as an aromatherapist depends on your level of expertise, the type of clientele you serve, and even the area of the country. In many of the larger cities and much of the West Coast, people are already more aware and accepting of alternative health therapies. In those areas, higher hourly rates will be more accepted. Where such therapies are practically unknown, lower rates will apply. Another consideration for the self-employed is that they must provide their own insurance and retirement plans and pay for their supplies and other business expenses.

If you have the determination, creativity, and initiative, you can find jobs that pay well. Some who run exclusive spas or develop their own lines of aromatherapy products are reported to earn $70,000 to $80,000 or more.

Aromatherapists who are primarily employed in other professions, such as massage therapists, chiropractors, cosmetologists, and nurses can expect to make the salaries that are average for their profession. Those professionals who use aromatherapy as a supportive therapy to their primary profession tend to have higher incomes than those who specialize in aromatherapy.

Work Environment

Aromatherapists work in a service-oriented environment, in which the main duty involves understanding and helping their clients. The surroundings are usually clean, peaceful, and pleasant. They work with very potent substances (strong essential oils), but most aromatherapists love the scents and the experience of the oils. They often spend a great deal of time on their feet. They sometimes work long or inconsistent hours, such as weekends and evenings, to accommodate their clients' needs.

Aromatherapists are people-oriented. They work with people and must be able to work well both individually and on teams. Those who are self-employed must be highly motivated and able to work alone. Aromatherapists who work in clinics, spas, hospitals, resorts, and other locations need to be good team players.

Outlook

Aromatherapy has been growing very rapidly. From 1996 to 1999, the number of students studying aromatherapy at one college increased almost 600 percent. Aromatherapy is just beginning to gather steam in the United States, and opportunities are increasing rapidly as public awareness of alternative therapies is increasing.

If we look at the status of the field in European and other countries, we may get a glimpse of the future of the field in the United States. In Great Britain and France, more doctors have embraced aromatherapy and these services are covered by major health plans. If we in the United States follow this lead, new doors will open in this field. In general, the outlook is very good for aromatherapy because of an overwhelming increase in public awareness and interest.

For More Information

NAHA is dedicated to the development of high standards of aromatherapy teaching and practice. It is currently developing a set of standards for aromatherapy, in an effort to provide guidelines for students and teachers.

National Association for Holistic Aromatherapy
836 Hanley Industrial Court
St. Louis, MO 63144
Tel: 888-ASK-NAHA or 314-963-2071
Web: http://www.naha.org

For information regarding state regulations for massage therapists and general information on therapeutic massage, contact:

American Massage Therapy Association
820 Davis Street, Suite 100
Evanston, IL 60201-4444
Tel: 847-864-0123
Web: http://www.amtamassage.org

Ayurvedic Doctors and Practitioners

Overview

Ayurvedic doctors and practitioners use theories and techniques developed thousands of years ago in India to bring people into physical, mental, emotional, and spiritual balance, thereby maintaining health, curing diseases, and promoting happiness and fulfillment. In the West, where Ayurveda is not an officially accepted and licensed form of medicine, only licensed medical doctors who are also thoroughly trained in Ayurveda can legally practice Ayurvedic medicine. They are Ayurvedic doctors. Licensed practitioners of paramedical professions, such as nutritionists, psychologists, naturopaths, massage therapists, and acupuncturists, may, if they are also trained in Ayurveda and use Ayurvedic techniques in their professional work, be called Ayurvedic practitioners. Any non-M.D. who practices the full range of Ayurvedic medicine in the West, however, is in danger of being seen as practicing medicine without a license, which is illegal.

History

The Vedas, which may be up to 5,000 years old, are the oldest and most important scriptures of Hinduism, which is the primary religion in India. The Sanskrit word *veda* means "knowledge," and the Vedas contain the knowledge and beliefs on which Hinduism is based. The Atharvaveda—the Veda that deals primarily with the practical aspects of life—contains chants, rites, and spells that are thought to enable believers to do such things as create love and goodwill among people, defeat enemies, and ensure success in agriculture. Most experts believe that the Atharvaveda is the basis of Ayurveda.

The word *Ayurveda* means "knowledge of life," and the oldest of the specifically Ayurvedic texts is the *Charaka Samhita*, which deals with internal medicine. That text was written in approximately 1000 BC, and it and more recent texts, such as the *Astanga Hridayam,* a compilation of Ayurvedic knowledge that was written in approximately AD 1000, provide Ayurvedic practitioners with the knowledge they need to help their patients.

Ayurvedic medicine is officially accepted in India, where approximately 80 percent of those who seek medical help go to Ayurvedic doctors. In its country of origin, Ayurveda has been substantially modernized, and it now includes many techniques and medications that originated in the West (although traditional doctors can still be found). In addition to ancient herbal formulas, for example, Indian Ayurvedic doctors often prescribe antibiotics. Indian doctors have not hesitated to discard certain of the older practices that are described in early texts, such as the use of leeches for bloodletting. In the West, however, some patients and practitioners utilize techniques that are now rarely used in India.

The Job

Ayurveda is a way of life rather than simply a system of healing. It is a holistic system, which means that it does not view physical health as something separate from spiritual health and mental health. An Ayurvedic doctor or practitioner treats the whole person, not simply the symptoms that a patient displays.

Ayurvedic doctors and practitioners base their treatments and recommendations on a complex body of beliefs. One of the most important beliefs in Ayurveda holds that everything in the universe is composed of one or more of the five elements: air, fire, earth, water, and ether (or space). These elements are concepts or qualities as much as they are actual entities. For example, anything that has the qualities that Ayurveda associates with fire is a manifestation of fire. A person's violent temper demonstrates the existence of fire within that person.

For the purposes of treating people, Ayurveda distills the concept of the five elements to three combinations of two elements. These are the *doshas,* which may be thought of as qualities or energies. The first dosha, Vata, is a combination of air and ether, with air predominating. The second dosha, Pitta, is a combination of fire and water, with fire predominating. The third dosha, Kapha, is a combination of water and earth, with water predominating. Every person is dominated by one or more doshas, although every person contains some element of all three. The unique combination of doshas that appears in a person is that person's *tridosha,* and that combination determines the person's constitution, or *prakriti.*

Because Ayurvedic theory holds that a person's nature and personality are based on his or her doshic makeup, or tridosha, the first thing that an Ayurvedic doctor or practitioner does when seeing a patient is to determine what that doshic makeup is. This is done by various means, including observation of physical qualities such as build, nails, lips, hair color, eye color, and skin type; taking the pulse in various locations; examination of the "nine doors," which are eyes, ears, nostrils, mouth, genitals, and anus; and questioning the patient about past history, present problems, goals, and so forth. After analyzing all this information, the practitioner determines which dosha or combination of doshas predominates in the patient's makeup.

Vata people tend to be extremely tall or extremely short and to have long fingers and toes. They are thin, have difficulty gaining weight, and have dark complexions and dry skin. The air element that predominates in their makeup makes them tend to be light, cold, and dry in various ways. They are often extremely creative, but their minds tend to flit from idea to idea, and they may be spacy and disorganized.

Pitta people, who are dominated by the fire element, are generally of medium build, and their fingers and toes are of medium length. They have little difficulty gaining or losing weight, and they are fair in complexion, with blond, light brown, or red hair. All redheads are said to have a significant amount of Pitta in their tridoshas. Pittas are quick to anger, can be forceful and domineering, and are highly organized. They make good engineers, accountants, and managers.

Kapha people, who are dominated by the water element, are generally large and well-built, with dark hair and oily skin. Their toes and fingers are short and thick. Kaphas often gain weight easily but have great physical stamina. They are usually calm people who avoid confrontation, but once they are angered, they hold a grudge. They like routine, tend not to be extremely creative, and are reliable.

Once the practitioner has determined the patient's tridosha and has ascertained what the patient's condition, problems, and desires are, he or she will create a program that will improve the patient's health and well-being. One of the most important methods that the practitioner will use is diet. If the patient's tridosha is out of balance, controlled to an extreme degree by one of the doshas, the practitioner may put together a diet that will decrease that dosha and/or increase the others, gradually and safely bringing the patient to a state of balance. Ayurvedic practitioners must therefore have a thorough knowledge of foods, traditional nutrition, and cooking.

Proper eating and good digestion are extremely important in Ayurveda, but Ayurvedic practitioners also use many other methods, among which are the techniques of *panchakarma,* which means "five actions." Panchakarma is a powerful set of cleansing practices that is ideally undertaken only under the guidance of an Ayurvedic doctor. The treatment varies by individual, but generally a patient must undergo one to seven days of preparation before the treatment begins. The preparation involves oil massage and steam baths, which sometimes include herbal treatments. After the body is sufficiently cleansed, the panchakarma may begin.

The first of the five practices is *vamana,* which involves removing excess Kapha from the stomach by inducing vomiting by gentle means. The second practice is *virechana,* which involves using laxatives to purge the body of excess Pitta. The third and fourth practices are both forms of *vasti,* or enema therapy, in which herbal preparations are used to remove Vata from the system. One form is relatively mild; the other is stronger. The fifth practice is *nasya,* which involves ingesting liquid or powdered substances through the nose. This practice is generally used to treat illnesses that affect the head and neck. It can take up to 30 days to complete the process of panchakarma.

There are many more aspects of Ayurvedic practice, and one of the most important things that doctors and practitioners do is advise patients regarding their lifestyle. They recommend various practices, such as cleaning the tongue daily, engaging in meditation, doing hatha yoga, and massaging the body with oils suitable for one's tridosha and the time of year. They may even advise patients regarding what kinds of clothes are best for them and where they will be most comfortable living.

Requirements

High School

The most important thing a high school student who wishes to become an Ayurvedic practitioner or doctor can do is learn as much as possible about health, medicine, science, and anatomy, just as a person who wants to become a Western medical doctor would. Courses in biology and chemistry are important. It will also be important to study the Hindu tradition and become familiar with Sanskrit terms. Studying Sanskrit, the language of the Vedas and the Ayurvedic texts, is a good idea, although it is not absolutely essential. Although Sanskrit is not offered in high schools, correspondence courses are available, and students in large cities may find Sanskrit courses in universities or may find teachers in an Indian community.

Postsecondary Training

Postsecondary training depends on the course the student wishes to take. To become a full-fledged Ayurvedic doctor in the West, a student must be trained as a medical doctor as well as in Ayurveda, which means getting a bachelor's degree, going to medical school, and completing an internship. According to Scott Gerson, M.D., a fully trained Ayurvedic doctor who runs the National Institute of Ayurvedic Medicine (NIAM), specializing in internal medicine or family practice is usually the best route for those who wish to become Ayurvedic doctors, although it is possible to combine other medical specialties with Ayurvedic practice in a beneficial way. Those who wish to combine Ayurveda with careers as nutritionists, psychologists, naturopaths, and so forth must complete the educational and training requirements for those specialties as well as study Ayurveda. It is not a good idea to go into business in a Western country simply as an expert in Ayurveda, since no licensing is available and doing so may leave you open to charges of practicing medicine without a license.

The single most important part of a doctor's or practitioner's Ayurvedic training is the completion of a rigorous course of study and practice. Naturally, a student who wishes to practice should select the most comprehensive course available. An excellent way to learn Ayurveda is to study at a good Indian institution and become a full-fledged Ayurvedic doctor in India. That kind of program typically takes five years to complete and also involves supervised practice afterward. Remember, though, that being licensed in India does not make it legal to practice as a doctor in the West. Alternatively, a student may study in the West, where various institutions offer Ayurvedic training. NIAM will offer a three-year program beginning in October of 1999. Beginning in 2000, NIAM will offer a four-year program, the most extensive in the United States.

Other Requirements

Ayurvedic practitioners and doctors work closely with their clients, so it is essential that they be able to gain their clients' or patients' trust, make them comfortable and relaxed, and communicate effectively enough with them to gather the information that they need in order to treat them effectively. It is unlikely that an uncommunicative person who is uncomfortable with people will be able to build a successful Ayurvedic practice. In addition, a practitioner must be comfortable making decisions and working alone.

Although some jobs are available in alternative health practices, most Ayurvedic doctors and practitioners have their own practices, and anyone who sets up shop will need to deal with the basic tasks and problems that all business owners face: advertising, accounting, taxes, legal requirements, and so forth. In addition, because Ayurveda is rooted in Hinduism, people whose religious beliefs are in conflict with Hinduism or who are uncomfortable with organized religion may be unwilling or unable to practice Ayurveda effectively.

Exploring

The best way to learn about Ayurveda is to speak with those who practice it. Call practitioners and ask to interview them. Find practitioners in your area if you can, but do not hesitate to contact people in other areas. There is no substitute for learning from those who actually do the work. Although many practitioners run one-person practices, it may be possible to find work of some kind with a successful practitioner or a clinic in your area, especially if you live in a large city.

You should also do as much reading as you can on the subject. Many books on Ayurveda are available. Also look for information on Ayurveda in magazines that deal with alternative medicine or Hinduism. You may also wish to read about traditional Oriental medicine (TOM), which is similar to Ayurveda in many ways.

Employers

For the most part, Ayurvedic practitioners work for themselves, although some teach in institutions and others work for alternative clinics. It is probably wise to assume that you are going to run your own business.

Starting Out

In addition to receiving training in medicine or in another professional field of your choice, you should begin by taking the best, most comprehensive Ayurvedic course of study you can find. After that, if you have not found an organization that you can work for, you should begin to practice on your own. You may rent an office or set up shop at home. Be sure to investigate the state and local laws that affect you.

A practitioner who runs his or her own business must be well-versed in basic business skills. Take courses in business or get advice from the local office of the Small Business Administration. Seek advice from people you know who run their own businesses. Your financial survival will depend on your business skills, so be sure that you are as well prepared as possible.

Advancement

Because most Ayurvedic doctors and practitioners work for themselves, advancement in the field is directly related to the quality of treatment they provide and their business skills. The best way to get ahead is to prove to the members of your community that you are skilled, honest, professional, and effective. Before you can be financially successful, there must be a strong demand for your services. When you have attained a high level of skill and your clients or patients are urging their friends to take their business to you, you will surely be financially successful.

Earnings

Generally, Ayurvedic doctors earn what most doctors in their fields of specialty earn. The situation is the same for practitioners, who generally earn what other people in their fields earn. It is probably safe to say that Ayurvedic practitioners on the low end make $20,000 per year and up, practitioners in more lucrative fields make between $35,000 and $60,000, and doctors earn amounts up to—and in some cases even more than—$150,000.

Work Environment

Ayurvedic practitioners usually work in their own homes or offices. Some practitioners may have office help, while others work alone. For this reason, they must be independent enough to work effectively on their own. Because they must make their clients comfortable in order to provide effective treatment, they generally try to make their workplaces as pleasant and relaxing as possible.

Outlook

Although no official government analysis of the future of Ayurveda has yet been conducted, it seems safe to say that the field is expanding much more rapidly than the average for all fields. Although science still views it with skepticism, Ayurveda has become relatively popular in a short period of time, largely because of the popularity of Deepak Chopra, an Ayurvedic expert who is also an M.D. It has certainly benefited from the popular acceptance of alternative medicine and therapies in recent years, particularly because it is a holistic practice that aims to treat the whole person rather than the symptoms of disease or discomfort. Because Western medicine is too often mechanical and dehumanizing, many people are looking for alternative forms of medicine.

For More Information

The AIVS provides on-site and correspondence training in Ayurveda, as well as courses in Sanskrit and other subjects that are of interest to Ayurvedic practitioners. It should be noted that correspondence courses do not qualify one as a practitioner, but they do prepare one for more in-depth training.

American Institute of Vedic Studies
PO Box 8357
Santa Fe, NM 87504-8357
Tel: 505-983-9385
Web: http://www.vedanet.com

The Ayurvedic Institute offers both on-site and correspondence courses in Ayurveda. Some of the organization's resources are available only to those who pay a membership fee.

The Ayurvedic Institute
11311 Menaul NE, Suite A
Albuquerque, NM 87112
Tel: 505-291-9698
Web: http://www.ayurveda.com

Deepak Chopra's Center does not offer training for practitioners, but it does offer courses for those who are interested in using Ayurveda in their own lives.

Chopra Center for Well Being
7640 Fay Avenue
La Jolla, CA 92037
Tel: 619-551-7788
Web: http://www.chopra.com

NIAM offers on-site training, sells correspondence courses, and sells Ayurvedic books and supplies. In October of 1999, it will offer a three-year training program in Ayurveda, and a four-year program will be available the following year.

National Institute of Ayurvedic Medicine
584 Milltown Road
Brewster, NY 10509
Tel: 888-246-6426
Web: http://www.niam.com

Certified Nurse-Midwives

Health Psychology Sociology	School Subjects
Communication/ideas Helping/teaching	Personal Skills
Bachelor's degree	Minimum Education Level
$21,580 to $45,840 to $70,100+	Salary Range
Required by all states	Certification or Licensing
Faster than the average	Outlook

Overview

Certified nurse-midwives are registered nurses who assist in family planning, pregnancy, and childbirth. They also provide routine health care for women. Certified nurse-midwives work in hospitals, with physicians in private practice, in freestanding birth centers or well-woman care centers, in women's clinics, and even in the homes of clients.

History

Women have been giving birth by "natural" methods for thousands of years, since pain medication, hospitals, and medical intervention were largely unavailable until recent years. Women gave birth at home, guided by other women who were designated assistants, or midwives. *Midwife* means "with woman," and early midwives, like today's professional certified nurse-midwives (CNMs), coached mothers-to-be through their pregnancy and labor. They helped women deliver their babies and taught new mothers how to care for their infants.

In the early 1900s, however, birth was transformed from a natural event into a technological marvel. New pain medications and medical procedures took birth into the 20th century, and childbearing moved from home to hospital. Back then, midwives practiced mainly in rural areas where doctors were unavailable, or where poorer women could not afford to deliver in a hospital.

Ironically, as these medically assisted births became more prevalent in America, professional midwifery became more regulated than it had been in the past. In the early 1920s, nurse Mary Breckenridge founded the Frontier Nursing Service in eastern Kentucky to bring medical services to people in areas too poor for hospitals, as well as to women who could not afford to have their babies delivered by a high-priced doctor. After completing her midwifery training in England, she made prenatal care an additional focus of her service.

Midwife care around the world was proving itself to be both low in cost and high in quality. The Maternity Association and the Lobenstine Clinic (both in New York) established the first U.S. midwifery school and graduated its first class in 1933. In the mid-1930s, the Frontier Nursing Service opened its own nurse-midwifery school, and it remains today the oldest continuing U.S. midwifery program.

During the next few decades, most women who were able to deliver in a hospital preferred the lull of pain medication and the perceived safety of the medical establishment, and midwifery remained a tool of poor and rural women. Pregnancy and childbirth were considered medical procedures best left in the hands of obstetricians and gynecologists. Both the medical community and the public have generally frowned upon midwifery in favor of doctors and hospitals.

Since the 1960s, however, this attitude has been changing as more women insist on more natural methods of giving birth. In 1968, the American College of Nurse-Midwives (ACNM), the premier midwife organization in the United States, was established. This creation of a nationally standardized entity to regulate midwife training and practice introduced midwifery as a positive, healthy, and safe alternative to hospital births. The nurse-midwife, officially known as a certified nurse-midwife (CNM), has gradually become accepted as a respected member of the health care teams involved with family planning, pregnancy, and labor.

A number of studies have indicated that babies delivered by nurse-midwives are less likely to experience low birth weights and other health complications than babies delivered by physicians. In fact, a recent study from the National Center for Health Statistics, Centers for Disease Control and Prevention indicates that the risk of death for the baby during birth was 19 percent lower for CNM-assisted deliveries than for physician-attended births.

The proven safety standards of births attended by nurse-midwives, the cost-effectiveness of a CNM-assisted pregnancy and labor, and the personal touch that many women get from their nurse-midwives will ensure that CNMs become vital links between traditional birthing practices and the high-tech worlds of today and tomorrow.

The Job

Nurse-midwives examine pregnant women and monitor the growth and development of fetuses. Typically a nurse-midwife is responsible for all phases of a normal pregnancy, including prenatal care, assisting during labor, and providing follow-up care. A certified nurse-midwife always works in consultation with a physician, who can be called upon should complications arise during pregnancy or childbirth. Nurse-midwives can provide emergency assistance to their patients while physicians are called. In most states, nurse-midwives are authorized to prescribe and administer medications. Many nurse-midwives provide the full spectrum of women's health care, including regular gynecological exams and well-woman care.

Not all midwives are certified nurse-midwives. Most states recognize other categories of midwives, including direct-entry (or licensed) midwives, certified professional midwives (CPMs), and lay (or empirical) midwives.

Direct-entry midwives are not required to be nurses in order to practice as midwives. They typically assist in home births or at birthing centers and are trained through a combination of formal education, apprenticeship, and self-education. Direct-entry midwives are legally recognized in 29 states that offer licensing, certification, or registration programs, and they perform most of the services of CNMs. Although they generally have professional relationships with physicians, hospitals, and laboratories to provide support and emergency services, few direct-entry midwives actually practice in medical centers.

Certified professional midwives (CPMs) must meet the basic requirements of the North American Registry of Midwives (NARM). Potential CPMs must pass a written examination and an assessment of their skills, and they must have proven training assisting in out-of-hospital births. NARM accepts various midwifery programs and practical apprenticeship as a basis for certification.

Lay midwives usually train by apprenticing with established midwives, although some may acquire formal education as well. Lay midwives are not certified or licensed, either because they lack the necessary experience and education or because they pursue nontraditional childbirth techniques.

Many lay midwives practice only as part of religious communities or specific ethnic groups, and typically assist only in home birth situations. Some states have made it illegal for lay midwives to charge for their services.

Since the education and certification standards for direct-entry midwives, certified professional midwives, and lay midwives vary from state to state, the rest of this article will deal only with certified nurse-midwives, who must complete a core nursing curriculum—as well as midwifery training—to become midwives. When the terms "nurse-midwife" and "midwife" are used in this article, certified nurse-midwife is implied.

Deborah Woolley has been a registered nurse since 1975 and has been practicing as a nurse-midwife since 1983. For Deborah, midwifery offered her the opportunity to have a positive impact on women's health care and childbirth experiences. "I started out as a nurse assigned to the labor and delivery unit. But I became frustrated with the type of care the women were getting," Deborah says. "You'll find that a lot among midwives. Most of the midwives I talk to can point to an event that was the straw that broke the camel's back, as it were—when they realized that they wanted to have more influence over the experience the woman is having. Midwifery's focus is on improving conditions for women and their families. In a way, midwifery is a radical departure from the old way of looking at pregnancy."

Deborah typically arrives at the hospital at 7:00 AM and spends the first hour or more seeing patients in postpartum—that is, women who have given birth the day or night before. At about 8:30 AM, Deborah goes down to the clinic to begin seeing other patients. "I work a combination of full days and half days during the week. On a half day, I'll see patients for four hours and work on paperwork for one hour. On a full day, I'll see patients for eight hours and work on paperwork for two hours," Deborah says. "But that doesn't mean I always leave exactly at five o'clock. At the clinic, we see everyone who shows up."

After Deborah meets a new patient, she'll spend an hour or so taking the patient's medical history, examining her, and getting her scheduled into the prenatal care system. "I also ask about a patient's life. I spend time with the patient and try to get to know her and what's going on in her life. It makes a big difference in the care she's provided. I think one of the things that makes midwives so effective is that they really get to know their patients."

An important part of a certified nurse-midwife's work is the education of patients. Nurse-midwives teach their patients about proper nutrition and fitness for healthy pregnancies and about different techniques for labor and delivery. Nurse-midwives also counsel their patients in the postpartum period about breast-feeding, parenting, and other areas concerning the health of mother and child. Nurse-midwives provide counseling on several other issues, including sexually transmitted diseases, spousal and child abuse, and social support networks. In some cases, this counseling may extend to family members of the soon-to-be or new mother, or even to older siblings of the family's newest addition. Deborah believes that this education is one of a midwife's key responsibilities. "I spend a lot of time teaching things like nutrition, the process of fetal development, and basic parenting skills. I'll refer patients to Lamaze classes. I'll also screen patients for family problems, such as violence in the home, and teach them how to get out of abusive situations," Deborah says. "In other words, I'll teach a patient anything she needs to know if she's pregnant. I try to empower women to take charge of their own health care and their own lives."

Apart from seeing patients, Deborah is also responsible for maintaining patient records. "I have to review lab results and ultrasounds and fill out birth certificates—things like that," she says. "There's a lot of writing involved, too. I have to document everything that I do with patients, including what I've done and how and why I've done it." This may include recording patient information, filing documents and patient charts, doing research to find out why a woman is having a particular problem, and consulting with physicians and other medical personnel. Many midwives build close relationships with their patients and try to be available for their patients at any time of the day or night.

Requirements

High School

In high school, you should begin preparing for a career as a nurse-midwife by taking a broad range of college preparatory courses, with a focus on science classes. Anatomy, biology, and chemistry will give you solid background information for what you will be studying in college. Additional classes in sociology and psychology will help you learn how to deal with a variety of patients from different ethnic and economic groups. English and business classes will teach you how to deal with the paperwork involved in any profession. Finally, you should consider learning foreign languages if you want to serve as a midwife to immigrant communities.

Postsecondary Training

All certified nurse-midwives begin their careers as registered nurses. In order to become a registered nurse, you will need to graduate from either a four-year bachelor's degree program in nursing or a two-year associate's degree program in nursing. After receiving a degree, you can apply for admission into an accredited certificate program in nurse-midwifery or an accredited master's degree program in nurse-midwifery.

With an associate's degree in nursing, you will be eligible for acceptance into a nurse-midwifery certificate program. A certificate program typically requires nine to twelve months of study. In order to be accepted into a master's degree program in nurse-midwifery, you must first earn your bachelor's degree in nursing. A master's degree program requires 16 to 24 months of study. Some master's degree programs also require one year of clinical experience in order to earn a nurse-midwife degree. In these programs, the prospective nurse-midwife is trained to provide primary care services, gynecological care, preconception and prenatal care, labor delivery and management, and postpartum and infant care.

Procedures that nurse-midwives are trained to perform include physical examinations, pap smears, and episiotomies. They may also repair incisions from cesarean sections, administer anesthesia, and prescribe medications. Nurse-midwives are trained to provide counseling on subjects such as nutrition, breastfeeding, and infant care. Nurse-midwives learn to provide both physical and emotional support to pregnant women and their families.

Certification or Licensing

After earning either a midwifery certificate from a nationally accredited nurse-midwifery program or a master's degree in midwifery, midwives are required to take a national examination administered by the American College of Nurse-Midwives (ACNM). Upon passing the exam, the new midwife achieves full endorsement as a medical professional, as well as the title "certified nurse-midwife." Those who have passed this examination are licensed to practice nurse-midwifery in all 50 states. Each state, however, has its own laws and regulations governing the activities and responsibilities of nurse-midwives.

Other Requirements

If you are interested in becoming a certified nurse-midwife, you will need skills that aren't necessarily taught in midwifery programs. Nurse-midwives need to enjoy working with people, learning about their patients' needs, and helping them through a very important life change. They should be sympathetic to the needs of their patients. They need to be independent and able to accept responsibility for their actions and decisions. Strong observation skills are key, as nurse-midwives must be tuned into their patient's needs during pregnancy and labor. Nurse-midwives also need to listen well and respond appropriately. They must communicate effectively with patients, family members, physicians, and other hospital staff, as well as insurance company personnel. Finally, nurse-midwives should be confident and composed, responding well in an emergency and keeping their patients calm.

Exploring

Volunteer work as a "candy striper" at your local hospital or clinic may put you in contact with nurse-midwives who can help you learn more about midwifery. You might also volunteer to visit and offer emotional support to laboring mothers-to-be at a hospital or freestanding birth center.

You may wish to contact a professional midwifery organization for more information about the field. These associations often publish journals or newsletters to keep members informed of new issues in midwifery. The better known organizations may have Web sites that can give you more information about midwifery in your area. A list of some organizations is at the end of this article.

Finally, young women may wish to see a nurse-midwife in lieu of a physician for their well-woman care. Although nurse-midwives are usually thought of in conjunction with pregnancy, many women use nurse-midwives as their primary medical contact from their teenage years through menopause.

Employers

Hospitals are the primary source of employment for certified nurse-midwives. Approximately 85 percent of the more than 6,000 nurse-midwives in the United States work in hospitals. They see patients and attend deliveries on hospital grounds and use hospital-owned equipment for examinations and other procedures. Additional medical personnel are always available for emergency situations. Most of the remaining nurse-midwives work in family planning clinics and other health care clinics and privately funded agencies. These nurse-midwives usually have relationships with specific hospitals and physicians in case of an emergency. Finally, some nurse-midwives operate their own clinics and birthing centers, while others work independently and specialize in home birth deliveries.

Starting Out

Deborah Woolley earned a bachelor's degree in nursing and then began her career as a nurse at a labor and delivery unit in a Texas hospital. While working, she attended graduate school and earned a master's degree in maternal child nursing. She then went to Chicago, where she began training as a nurse-midwife. "After earning my nurse-midwifery degree," Deborah says, "I heard there were openings at Cook County Hospital here in Chicago. So I applied for a job there. What I liked about Cook County was that they continued to train me while I was working. They gave me assertiveness training and training in urban health issues."

Like Deborah, most certified nurse-midwives finish their formal education in nursing and midwifery before beginning work. They usually have some opportunities to work with patients as a student. Beginning midwives may also intern at a hospital or clinic to fulfill class requirements.

Certified nurse-midwives can begin their careers in various ways. Some may move from an internship to a full-time job when they complete their education requirements at a certain facility. Others may seek out a position through a professional midwifery organization or try for a job at a specific location that interests them. Finally, some nurse-midwives begin by working as nurses in other areas of health care and then move into midwifery as opportunities become available.

Advancement

With experience, a nurse-midwife can advance into a supervisory role or into an administrative capacity at a hospital, family planning clinic, birthing center, or other facility. Many nurse-midwives, like Deborah Woolley, choose to continue their education and complete Ph.D. programs. With a doctorate, a nurse-midwife can do research or teaching. "I spent four-and-a-half years at Cook County while I was working on my Ph.D.," Deborah says. "From there I was recruited to Colorado to head up the midwifery unit at a hospital there. After six years as a director in Colorado, I learned that the director's position here at UIC was open, and I jumped at the chance to come back to Chicago."

Nurse-midwives with advanced degrees may choose to move away from the day-to-day patient care and write for journals or magazines. They may also lean more towards the research aspects of prenatal care and obstetrics. Finally, nurse-midwives may prefer to apply their experience and education and move toward other areas of medicine or hospital administration.

Earnings

According to the 1998-99 *Occupational Outlook Handbook*, nurse-midwives earned about $70,100—with the middle 50 percent earning between $59,300 and $75,700—per year in 1996. Although this would put certified nurse-midwives among the highest paid nursing professionals, other salary estimates are more conservative. Starting salaries for beginning nurse-midwives can range from $21,580 to around $45,000 per year, depending on the place of employment; those working for large hospitals tend to earn more that those working for small hospitals, clinics, and birthing centers. The most experienced nurse-midwives, including those in supervisory, director, and administrative positions, can earn much more. Salaries also vary according to the region of the country and whether the employing facility is private or public.

Nurse-midwives generally enjoy a good benefits package, although these too can vary widely depending on employer. CNMs working in hospitals or well-established clinics or birthing centers usually receive a full complement of benefits, including medical coverage, paid sick time, and holiday and vacation pay. They may also be able to work a more flexible schedule to accommodate family or personal obligations.

Work Environment

Nurse-midwives who work in hospitals or as part of a physician's practice work indoors in clean, professional surroundings. Although most nurse-midwives perform checkups and routine visits alone with their patients, a number of other health care professionals are on hand in case the midwife has a question or needs assistance in an emergency. Nurse-midwives often consult with doctors, medical insurance representatives, family members of their patients, as well as other midwives in order to determine the best care routine for the women they serve.

In a hospital, CNMs usually wear professional clothing, a lab coat, and comfortable shoes to allow for plenty of running around during the day. They often wear hospital scrubs during delivery. In a free-standing birth center, the nurse-midwives may have a more casual dress code but still maintain a professional demeanor.

Midwives try to make their offices and birthing areas as calm and as reassuring as possible so their patients feel comfortable during checkups and delivery. Soft music may play in the background, or the waiting area may be decorated like a nursery and filled with parenting magazines.

Although most nurse-midwives work a 40-hour week, these hours may not reflect the typical nine-to-five day, since babies are delivered at all hours of the day and night. Many hospitals or clinics offer nurse-midwives a more flexible schedule in exchange for having the CNM "on-call" for births.

Finally, although there are no gender requirements in the profession, nurse-midwifery is a field dominated by women. Well over 98 percent of CNMs in the United States are female. Women have traditionally helped each other through pregnancy and delivery. Just as women who became doctors 100 years ago had to overcome many barriers, men considering entering midwifery should be prepared for hurdles of their own.

Outlook

The number of nurse-midwifery jobs is expected to grow faster than the average for all occupations through 2006, as nurse-midwives gain a reputation as an integral part of the health care community. Currently, there are more positions than there are CNMs to fill them. This situation is expected to continue for the near future.

There are two factors driving the demand for nurse-midwives. The first element is the growth of interest in natural childbearing techniques among women. The number of midwife-assisted births has risen dramatically since the 1970s. Some women have been attracted to midwifery because of studies that indicate natural childbirth is more healthful for mother and child than doctor-assisted childbirth. Other women have been attracted to midwifery because it emphasizes the participation of the entire family in prenatal care and labor.

The second factor in the growing demand for nurse-midwives is economic. As society moves toward managed care programs and the health care community emphasizes cost-effectiveness, midwifery should increase in popularity. This is because the care provided by nurse-midwives costs substantially less than the care provided by obstetricians and gynecologists. If the cost advantage of midwifery continues, more insurers and health maintenance organizations will probably direct patients to certified nurse-midwives for care.

For More Information

ACNM is the largest and most widely known midwifery organization in the United States. For more information about the midwife certification process, contact:

American College of Nurse-Midwives
818 Connecticut Avenue, NW, Suite 900
Washington, DC 20006
Tel: 202-728-9860
Web: http://www.midwife.org/ or http://www.acnm.org/

MANA can give you information about all types of midwifery (not just CNM):

Midwives Alliance of North America
Tel: 888-923-MANA (6262)
Web: http://www.mana.org/

Chiropractors

School Subjects
Biology
Chemistry
English

Personal Skills
Mechanical/manipulative
Technical/scientific

Work Environment
Primarily indoors
Primarily one location

Minimum Education Level
Medical degree

Salary Range
$39,000 to $88,500 to $102,500

Certification or Licensing
Required by all states

Outlook
Faster than the average

Overview

Chiropractors, or *doctors of chiropractic,* are health care professionals who practice the holistic, drugless, healing art of chiropractic. They emphasize health maintenance and disease prevention through proper nutrition, exercise, posture, stress management, and care of the spine and the nervous system. In 1996, there were around 44,000 chiropractors in the United States. Most work in solo practice, in partnerships, or in health care clinics.

Because of its emphasis on health maintenance, the whole person, and natural healing, it is considered an alternative health care approach. At the same time, chiropractic has more of the advantages enjoyed by the medical profession than does any other alternative health care field: chiropractic has licensure requirements, accredited training institutions, a growing scientific research base, and insurance reimbursement.

History

Although chiropractic as we know it is just over 100 years old, spinal manipulation dates back to ancient civilizations. Reports of manipulative therapy were recorded in China as early as 2700 BC. Hippocrates, the "father of medicine," used spinal manipulation around the 4th century BC to reposition vertebrae and to heal other ailments. Galen, a renowned Greek physician who practiced in Rome during the 2nd century AD, used spinal manipulation. Ambroise Paré, who is sometimes called the "father of surgery," used it in France in the 16th century. These "bone-setting" techniques were passed down through through the centuries through family tradition. They can be found in the folk medicine of many countries. In 1843, Dr. J. Evans Riadore, a physician, studied the irritation of spinal nerves and recommended spinal manipulation as a treatment.

Daniel D. Palmer, an American, founded the system of chiropractic in 1895. He also coined the term *chiropractic*. Palmer believed that deviations of the spinal column, or subluxations, were the cause of practically all disease and that chiropractic adjustment was the cure. Like many others who have tried to change the practice of medicine, Dr. Palmer encountered strong opposition from the medical establishment. He and other early chiropractors were imprisoned for practicing medicine without a license. In spite of the hardships, he and his followers persevered because of the success of their treatments in alleviating pain and promoting health. Their treatments at times had exceptionally positive results.

In spite of their successful work and a growing number of supporters, chiropractors were attacked by the medical establishment because they had little scientific research to support their claims. In the 1970s, Dr. Chang Ha Suh, Ph.D., a Korean immigrant who was working at the University of Colorado, had the courage to conduct studies that provided extensive scientific research related to chiropractic. Since then, numerous important studies have added to the research and to the credibility of chiropractic.

Today chiropractic is the third largest primary health care profession in the United States. Many good schools of chiropractic exist, and doctors of chiropractic are licensed in all 50 states and the District of Columbia. Chiropractic is one of the fastest growing health care professions in the country.

The Job

Chiropractors are trained primary health care providers, much like medical physicians. Chiropractors focus on the maintenance of health and disease prevention. In addition to symptoms, they consider each patient's nutrition, work, stress levels, exercise habits, posture, and so on. Chiropractors treat people of all ages—from children to senior citizens. They see both women and men. Doctors of chiropractic most frequently treat conditions such as backache, disc problems, sciatica, and whiplash. They also care for people with headaches, respiratory disorders, allergies, digestive disturbances, elevated blood pressure, and many other common ailments. Some specialize in areas such as sports medicine or nutrition. Chiropractors do not utilize drugs or surgery. If they determine that drugs or surgery are needed, they refer the individual to another professional who can meet those needs.

Doctors of chiropractic look for causes of disorders of the spine. They consider the spine and the nervous system to be vitally important to the health of the individual. Chiropractic teaches that problems in the spinal column (backbone) affect the nervous system and the body's natural defense mechanisms and are the underlying causes of many diseases. Chiropractors use a special procedure called a "spinal adjustment" to try to restore the spine to its natural healthy state. They believe this will also have an effect on the individual's total health and well-being.

On the initial visit, doctors of chiropractic meet with the patient and take a complete medical history before beginning treatment. They ask questions about all aspects of the person's life to help determine the nature of the illness. Events in the individual's past that may seem unrelated or unimportant may be significant to the chiropractor.

After the consultation and the case history, chiropractors perform a careful physical examination. The examination may include laboratory tests. When necessary, they use X rays to help locate the source of patients' difficulties. Doctors of chiropractic study the X rays for more than just a fracture or signs of disease. X rays are the only means of seeing the outline of the spinal column. Chiropractors are trained to observe whether the structural alignment of the spinal column is normal or abnormal.

Once they have made a diagnosis, chiropractic physicians use a variety of natural approaches to help restore the individual to health. The spinal adjustment is the treatment for which chiropractic is most known. During this procedure, patients usually lie on a specially designed adjusting table. Chiropractic physicians generally use their hands to manipulate the spine. They apply pressure and use specialized techniques of manipulation that are designed to help the affected areas of the spine. Doctors of chiropractic must know many sophisticated techniques of manipulation, and they spend countless hours learning to properly administer spinal adjustments. Chiropractic treatments must often be repeated over the course of several visits. The number of treatments needed varies greatly.

In addition to the spinal adjustment, chiropractic physicians may use "physiologic therapeutics" to relieve symptoms. These are drugless natural therapies, such as light, water, electrical stimulation, massage, heat, ultrasound, and biofeedback. Chiropractors also make suggestions about diet, rest, exercise, and support of the afflicted body part. They may recommend routines for the patient to do at home to maintain and improve the results of the manipulation.

Chiropractors pay special attention to lifestyle factors, such as nutrition and exercise. They believe the body has an innate ability to remain healthy if it has the proper ingredients. Doctors of chiropractic propose that the essential ingredients include clean air, water, proper nutrition, rest, and a properly functioning nervous system. Their goal is to maintain the health and well-being of the whole person. In this respect they have been practicing for many years what has recently become known as "health maintenance."

Chiropractors who are in private practice and some who work as group practitioners also have responsibility for running their businesses. They must promote their practices and develop their patient base. They are responsible for keeping records on their patients and for general bookkeeping. Sometimes they hire and train employees. In larger practices or clinics, chiropractic assistants or office managers usually perform these duties.

Requirements

High School

To become a doctor of chiropractic (DC), you will have to study a minimum of six to seven years after high school. Preparing for this profession is just as demanding as preparing to be a medical doctor, and the types of courses you will need are also similar. Science classes, such as biology, chemistry, physics, and psychology will prepare you for medical courses in college. English, speech, drama, and debate can sharpen the communication skills that are essential for this profession. Math, business, and computer classes can help you get ready to run a private practice.

Postsecondary Training

Most chiropractic colleges require at least two years of undergraduate study before you can enroll. Some require a bachelor's degree. In 1997, 16 institutions in the U.S. had chiropractic programs that were accredited by the Council on Chiropractic Education. Find out which chiropractic colleges interest you and learn about their requirements. Selecting chiropractic schools well in advance will allow you to structure your undergraduate study to meet the requirements of the schools of your choice. Some chiropractic colleges provide opportunities for prechiropractic study and bachelor's degree programs. In general, you need course work in biology, communications, English, chemistry, physics, psychology, and social sciences or humanities. Contact the national professional associations listed at the end of this article for information about schools and their requirements.

Upon completing the required undergraduate work and enrolling in a chiropractic college, you can expect to take an array of science and medical courses, such as anatomy, pathology, and microbiology. During the first two years of most chiropractic programs you will spend most of your time in the classroom or the laboratory. The last two years generally focus on courses in spinal adjustments. Most chiropractic students spend more than 500 hours learning to adjust. During this time, potential chiropractors also train in outpatient clinics affiliated with the college. Upon successful completion of the six- or seven-year professional degree program, you will receive the degree of Doctor of Chiropractic (DC).

Certification or Licensing

All 50 states and the District of Columbia require that chiropractors pass a state board examination to obtain a license to practice. Educational requirements and types of practice for which a chiropractor may be licensed vary from state to state. Most state boards recognize academic training only in chiropractic colleges accredited by the Council on Chiropractic Education. In addition to the state board examination, several states require that chiropractors pass a basic science examination. Most state boards will accept the National Board of Chiropractic Examiners' test given to fourth-year chiropractic students in place of a state exam. Most states require that chiropractors take continuing education courses each year to keep their licenses.

Other Requirements

Perhaps the most important personal requirement for any health care professional is the desire to help people and to promote wholeness and health. To be a successful chiropractor, you need good listening skills, empathy, and understanding. As a doctor of chiropractic, you will also need a good business sense and the ability to work independently. Especially sharp observational skills are essential in order for you to recognize physical abnormalities. Good hand dexterity is necessary to perform the spinal adjustments and other manipulations. However, you do not need unusual strength.

Exploring

If you are interested in becoming a chiropractor, there are many ways to start preparing right now. Join all the science clubs you can, design projects, and participate in science fairs. To develop interviewing and communication skills, you might join the school newspaper staff and ask for interview assignments. Learn to play chess or try to solve mystery stories to increase your powers of observation. Take up an instrument, such as the piano, guitar, or violin, to improve your manual dexterity. Learning to give massages is another way to increase manual dexterity.

Contact the chiropractic professional associations and ask about their student programs. Check out the Internet for bulletin boards or forums related to chiropractic and other areas of health care. Volunteer at a hospital or nursing home to gain experience working with those in need of medical care.

If there is a doctor of chiropractic or a clinic in your area, ask to visit and talk to a chiropractor. Make an appointment for a chiropractic examination so you can experience what it is like. You may even find a part-time or summer job in a chiropractic office.

Employers

A newly licensed doctor of chiropractic might find a salaried position in a chiropractic clinic or with an experienced chiropractor. Other salaried positions can be found in traditional hospitals, in hospitals that specialize in chiropractic treatment, or in alternative health care centers and clinics. About 70 percent of the doctors of chiropractic in the United States are in private practice. Most maintain offices in a professional building with other specialists or at their own clinics.

Chiropractors practice throughout the United States. Jobs in clinics, hospitals, and alternative health care centers may be easier to find in larger cities that have the population to support them. However, most doctors of chiropractic choose to work in small communities. Chiropractors tend to remain near chiropractic institutions, and this has resulted in higher concentrations of chiropractic practices in those geographical areas.

Starting Out

The placement offices of chiropractic colleges have information about job openings in the profession, and they may be able to help with job placement. As a newly licensed chiropractor, you might begin working in a clinic or in an established practice with another chiropractor on a salary or income-sharing basis. This would give you a chance to start practicing without the major financial investment of equipping an office. It is sometimes possible to purchase the practice of a chiropractor who is retiring or moving. This is usually easier than starting a new solo practice because the purchased practice will already have patients. However, some newly licensed practitioners do go straight into private practice.

Chiropractic colleges are good sources of information about setting up a practice. The national chiropractic associations and professional publications may list job openings. Go to meetings of national and state professional associations. These are excellent opportunities to get to know professionals in the field. Networking is an important way to learn about job openings.

Advancement

As with many other professions, advancement in chiropractic usually means building a larger practice. A chiropractor who starts out as a salaried employee in a large practice may eventually become a partner in the practice. Chiropractors also advance their careers by building their clientele and setting up their own group practices. They sometimes buy the practices of retiring practitioners to add to their own practices.

Another avenue for advancement is specialization. Chiropractors specialize in areas such as neurology, sports medicine, or diagnostic imaging (X ray). As the demand for chiropractors is growing, more are advancing their careers through teaching at chiropractic institutions or conducting research. A few doctors of chiropractic become executives with state or national organizations.

Earnings

According to the 1997 Statistical Survey of the American Chiropractic Association (ACA), the average gross income for chiropractic physicians was $228,236 in 1996. Mean practice expenses were $133,349, which left an average individual net income of $86,519. The report indicated that net incomes tend to increase during the first 20 years of practice. After that, there is a slight decline.

The ACA survey showed that chiropractors who were employed by someone else had the lowest net earnings ($38,968). Those who worked in private practice tended to have lower incomes than those in group or partnership practice ($84,228 versus $102,426). There is usually a strong correlation between number of hours worked and income.

Work Environment

Chiropractic physicians work in clean, quiet, comfortable offices. Most solo practitioners and group practices have an office suite. The suite generally has a reception area. In clinics, several professionals may share this area. The suite also contains examining rooms and treatment rooms. In a clinic where several professionals work, there are sometimes separate offices for the individual professionals. Most chiropractors have chiropractic assistants and a secretary or office manager. Those who are in private practice or partnerships need to have good business skills and self-discipline to be successful.

Doctors of chiropractic who work in clinics, hospitals, universities, or professional associations need to work well in a group environment. They will frequently work under supervision or in a team with other professionals. Chiropractors may have offices of their own, or they may share offices with team members, depending on their work and the facility. In these organizations, the physical work environment varies, but it will generally be clean and comfortable. Because they are larger, these settings may be noisier than the smaller practices.

Most chiropractors work about 42 hours per week, although many put in longer hours. Larger organizations may determine the hours of work, but chiropractors in private practice can set their own. Evening and weekend hours are often scheduled to accommodate patients' needs.

Outlook

The demand for doctors of chiropractic is expected to grow faster than the average through the year 2006. Many areas have a shortage of chiropractors. Public interest in alternative health care is growing. Many health-conscious individuals are attracted to chiropractic because it is natural, drugless, and surgery-free. Because of their holistic, personal approach to health care, chiropractors are increasingly seen as primary physicians, especially in rural areas. The average life span is increasing, and so are the numbers of older people in this country. The elderly frequently have more structural and mechanical difficulties, and the growth of this segment of the population will increase the demand for doctors of chiropractic.

More insurance policies and HMOs now cover chiropractic services, but this still varies according to the insurer. As a result of these developments in HMO and insurance coverage, chiropractors receive more referrals for treatment of injuries that result from accidents.

While the demand for chiropractic is increasing, college enrollments are also growing. New chiropractors may find increasing competition in geographic areas where other practitioners are already located. Because of the high cost of equipment such as X ray and other diagnostic tools, group practices with other chiropractors or related health care professionals are likely to provide more opportunity for employment or for purchasing a share of a practice.

For More Information

For general information, and a career kit, contact:

American Chiropractic Association
1701 Clarendon Boulevard
Arlington, VA 22209
Tel: 800-986-4636
Web: http://www.amerchiro.org

For information on educational requirements and accredited colleges, contact:

Council on Chiropractic Education
7975 North Hayden Road, Suite A-210
Scottsdale, AZ 85258
Tel: 602-443-8877

For information on student membership and member chiropractors in your area, contact:

International Chiropractors Association
1110 North Glebe Road, Suite 1000
Arlington, VA 22201
Tel: 800-423-4690
Web: http//www.chiropractic.org

For a list of chiropractic colleges in Canada, contact:

Canadian Chiropractic Association
1396 Eglinton Avenue West
Toronto, ON M6C 2E4 Canada

Creative Arts Therapists

Art Music Theater/Dance	School Subjects
Artistic Helping/teaching	Personal Skills
Master's degree	Minimum Education Level
$19,500 to $26,000 to $42,000+	Salary Range
Required by all states	Certification or Licensing
Faster than the average	Outlook

Overview

Creative arts therapists treat and rehabilitate people with mental, physical, and emotional disabilities. They use the creative processes of music, art, dance/movement, drama, psychodrama, and poetry in their therapy sessions to determine the underlying causes of some problems and to help patients achieve therapeutic goals. Creative arts therapists usually specialize in one particular type of therapeutic activity. The specific objectives of the therapeutic activities vary according to the needs of the patient and the setting of the therapy program.

History

Creative arts therapy programs are fairly recent additions to the health care field. Although many theories of mental and physical therapy have existed for centuries, it has been only in the last 70 years or so that health care professionals have truly realized the healing powers of music, art, dance, and other forms of artistic self-expression.

Art therapy is based on the idea that people who can't discuss their problems with words must have another outlet for self-expression. In the early 1900s, psychiatrists began to look more closely at their patients' artwork, realizing that there could be links between the emotional or psychological illness and the art. Sigmund Freud even did some preliminary research into the artistic expression of his patients.

In the 1930s, art educators discovered that children often expressed their thoughts better with pictures and role-playing than they did through verbalization. Children often don't know the words they need to explain how they feel, or how to make their needs known to adults. Researchers began to look into art as a way to treat children who were traumatized by abuse, neglect, illness, or other physical or emotional disabilities.

During and after World War II, the Department of Veterans Affairs (VA) developed and organized various art, music, and dance activities for patients in VA hospitals. These activities had a dramatic effect on the physical and mental well being of the World War II veterans, and creative arts therapists began to help treat and rehabilitate patients in other health care settings.

Because of early breakthroughs with children and veterans, the number of arts therapists has increased greatly over the past few decades, and the field has expanded to include drama, psychodrama, and poetry, as well as the more traditional music, art, and dance. Today creative arts therapists work with diverse populations of patients in a wide range of facilities, and they focus on the specific needs of a vast spectrum of disorders and disabilities. Colleges and universities offer degree programs in many types of therapies, and national associations for registering and certifying creative arts therapists work to monitor training programs and to ensure the professional integrity of the therapists working in the various fields.

The Job

Similar to dreaming, creative arts therapy taps into the subconscious and gives people a mode of expression in an uncensored environment. This is important because before patients can begin to heal, they must first identify their feelings. Once they recognize their feelings, they can begin to develop an understanding of the relationship between their feelings and their behavior.

The main goal of a creative arts therapist is to improve the patient's physical, mental, and emotional health. Before they begin any treatment, they meet with a team of other health care professionals. After determining the strength, limitations, and interests of their patient, they create a program to promote positive change and growth in the patient. The creative arts therapist continues to confer with the other health care workers as the program progresses, and alters the program according to the patient's progress. How these goals are reached depends on the unique specialty of the therapist in question.

"It's like sitting in the woods waiting for a fawn to come out." That is how Barbara Fish, Director of Activity Therapy for the Illinois Department of Mental Health and Developmental Disabilities, Chicago Metropolitan and Adolescent Services, describes her experience as she waits patiently for a sexually abused patient to begin to trust her. The patient is extraordinarily frightened because of the traumatic abuse she has suffered. This may be the first time in the patient's life that she is in an environment of acceptance and support. It may take months or even years before the patient begins to trust the therapist, "come out of the woods," and begin to heal.

In some cases, especially when the patients are adolescents, they may have become so detached from their feelings that they can physically act out without consciously knowing the reasons for their behavior. This detachment from their emotions creates a great deal of psychological pain. With the help of a creative arts therapist, patients can begin to communicate their subconscious feelings both verbally and nonverbally. They can express their emotions in a variety of ways without having to name them.

Creative arts therapists work with all age groups: young children, adolescents, adults, and senior citizens. They can work in individual, group, or family sessions. The approach of the therapist, however, depends on the specific needs of the patient or group. For example, if a patient is feeling overwhelmed by too many options or stimuli, the therapist may give him or her only a plain piece of paper and a pencil to work with that day.

Barbara Fish has three ground rules for her art therapy sessions with disturbed adolescents: respect yourself, respect other people, and respect property. The therapy groups are limited to five patients per group. She begins the session by asking each person in the group how he or she is feeling that day. By carefully listening to their responses, a theme may emerge that will determine the direction of the therapy. For example, if anger is reoccurring in their statements, Barbara may ask them to draw a line down the center of a piece of paper. On one side, she will ask them to draw how anger looks and on the other side how feeling sad looks. Then, once the drawing is complete, she will ask them to compare the two pictures and see that their anger may be masking their feelings of sadness, loneliness, and disappointment. As patients begin to recognize their true feelings, they develop better control of their behavior.

To reach their patients, creative arts therapists can use a variety of mediums, including visual art, music, dance, drama, or poetry or other kinds of creative writing. Creative arts therapists usually specialize in a specific medium, becoming a music therapist, drama therapist, dance therapist, art therapist, or poetry therapist. "In my groups we use poetry and creative writing," Barbara explains. "We do all kinds of things to get at what is going on at an unconscious level."

Music therapists use musical lessons and activities to improve a patient's self-confidence and self-awareness, to relieve states of depression, and to improve physical dexterity. For example, a music therapist treating a patient with Alzheimer's might play songs from the patient's past in order to stimulate long- and short-term memory, soothe feelings of agitation, and increase sense of reality.

Art therapists use art in much the same manner. The art therapist may encourage and teach patients to express their thoughts, feelings, and anxieties via sketching, drawing, painting, or sculpting. Art therapy is especially helpful in revealing patterns of domestic abuse in families. Children involved in such a situation may depict scenes of family life with violent details or portray a certain family member as especially frightening or threatening.

Dance/movement therapists develop and conduct dance/movement sessions to help improve physical, mental, and emotional health of their patients. Dance and movement therapy is also used as a way of assessing a patient's progress toward reaching therapeutic goals.

There are other types of creative arts therapists as well. *Drama therapists* use role-playing, pantomime (the telling of a story by the use of expressive body or facial movements), puppetry, improvisation, and original scripted dramatization to evaluate and treat patients. *Poetry therapists* and *bibliotherapists*, use the written and spoken word to treat patients.

Requirements

High School

A high school diploma or GED equivalent is mandatory to become a creative arts therapist. Depending on what type of creative arts therapy you might wish to pursue, you should become as proficient as possible with the methods and tools of the trade. For example, if you want to become involved in music therapy, you need to become familiar with musical instruments as well as music theory. A good starting point for a music therapist is to study piano or guitar. It is important that high school students wishing to become creative arts therapists begin studying any applicable art forms as soon as possible. When therapists work with patients they must be able to concentrate completely on the patient rather than on learning how to use tools or techniques.

In addition to courses such as drama, art, music, and English, students should consider taking an introductory class in psychology. Also, students should take a communication class to begin to gain an understanding of the various ways people communicate, both verbally and nonverbally.

Postsecondary Training

To become a creative arts therapist one must have earned at least a bachelor's degree, usually in the area in which one wishes to specialize. However, to be accredited, many nationally recognized associations require a graduate degree from a university with an accredited program. For instance, the American Association for Art Therapy requires a master's degree for accreditation.

Accredited graduate programs for creative arts therapists vary according to the discipline pursued. For example, graduate programs in art therapy require the applicant to submit a portfolio of original artwork. The portfolio should demonstrate a high level of competence with working with art materials, although not necessarily a great degree of talent.

Once accepted into a program, arts therapy students undergo rigorous classroom instruction that includes at least 15 semester hours of study in studio art and 12 semester hours of psychology. It is a requirement that these hours of study be completed within a year of beginning the program. In addition to class work, student must participate in 600 hours of supervised arts therapy practice, half of which is in individual sessions and half in group sessions. Finally, the core curriculum includes 21 graduate credit hours, which the student must complete within two years or four full-time semesters. Requirements in graduate programs for most of the other areas of creative arts therapy are similar to those for arts therapists.

Certification or Licensing

The nationally recognized association specific to their field of choice must certify most creative arts therapists. For instance, certification by the Art Therapy Credentials Board, Inc. (ATCB) is a two-part process. First, to become registered, the ATCB will review the applicant's documentation of graduate education and postgraduate supervised experience. Once the arts therapist is registered, he or she must pass a written examination administered by the ATCB to become board certified. To retain this status, therapists must continue their education.

Certification for most other creative arts therapies also requires passing a national examination. For example, a music therapist must pass an exam administered by the Certification Board for Music Therapists. The examination tests competence in individual skills and knowledge, and the practical application of professional music therapy.

Many registered creative arts therapists also receive additional licenses as social workers, educators, mental health professionals, or marriage and family therapists. They are also often members of other professional associations, including the American Psychological Association, the American Association of Marriage and Family Therapists, and the American Counseling Association.

Other Requirements

Creative arts therapists should have a strong desire to help others seek positive change in their lives. All types of creative arts therapists must be able to work well with other people—both patients and other health professionals—in the development and implementation of therapy programs. They must have the patience and the stamina to teach and practice therapy with patients for whom progress is often very slow because of their various physical and emotional disorders. A therapist must always keep in mind that even a tiny amount of progress might be extremely significant for some patients and their families. A good sense of humor is also a valuable trait for someone working in the field.

Exploring

There are many ways to explore the possibility of a career as a creative arts therapist. Students can write to professional associations for information on therapy careers. They can talk with people working in the creative arts therapy field and perhaps arrange to observe a creative arts therapy session. To see if they would be happy working in the field, students may seek part-time or summer jobs or volunteer at a hospital, clinic, nursing home, or any of a number of health care facilities.

A summer job as an aide at a camp for disabled children, for example, may help provide insight into the nature of creative arts therapy, including both its rewards and demands. Such experience can be very valuable in deciding if you are suited to the inherent frustrations of a therapy career.

Employers

Creative arts therapists usually work as members of an interdisciplinary health care team that may include physicians, nurses, social workers, psychiatrists, and psychologists. Although often employed in hospitals, therapists also work in rehabilitation centers, nursing homes, day treatment facilities, shelters for battered women, pain and stress management clinics, substance abuse programs, hospices, and correctional facilities. Others maintain their own private practices. Many creative arts therapists work with children in grammar and high schools, either as therapists or art teachers. Some arts therapists teach or conduct research in the creative arts at colleges and universities.

Starting Out

After earning a bachelor's degree in a particular field, potential creative arts therapists should complete their certification, which may include an internship or assistantship. Unpaid training internships often can lead to a first job in the field. Graduates can utilize the placement office at their college or university to help them find positions in the creative arts therapy field. Many professional associations also compile lists of job openings to assist their members.

Creative arts therapists who are new to the field might consider doing volunteer work at a nonprofit community organization, correctional facility, or other neighborhood association to gain some practical experience. Therapists who want to start their own practice can host group therapy sessions in their home. Creative arts therapists may also wish to associate themselves with other members of the alternative health care field in order to gain experience and build a client base.

Advancement

As therapists gain more experience, they can move into supervisory, administrative, or teaching positions. Often, the supervision of interns can resemble a therapy session. The interns will discuss their feelings and ask any questions that they may have regarding their work with patients. How did they handle their patients? What were the reactions to what their patients said or did? What could they be doing to help their patients more? The supervising therapist helps the interns become competent creative arts therapists.

Many therapists have represented the profession internationally. Barbara Fish was invited to present her paper, "Art Therapy with Children and Adolescents," at the University of Helsinki. Additionally, Barbara spoke in Finland at a three-day workshop exploring the use and effectiveness of arts therapy with children and adolescents. Raising the public and professional awareness of creative arts therapy is an important concern for many therapists.

Earnings

Because creative arts therapies are very broad in nature and are often used in conjunction with other treatments, it is difficult to estimate exact salary ranges for each subset (music therapists, drama therapists, etc.). As noted in the 1998-99 *Occupational Outlook Handbook,* an American Therapeutic Recreation Association survey indicates that recreational therapists (who have many of the same duties and qualifications as creative arts therapists) earned about $33,000 in 1996. Those in consultant, supervisory, administrative, and teaching positions in the field earned around $42,000 in 1996. Those working in government positions earned about $39,400 in 1997. Therapists just starting out in the field generally earn considerably less, usually between $20,000 and $26,000 per year.

Creative arts therapists who run their own practices may earn less because they have to cover their own business upkeep costs, in addition to advertising and insurance. Professional therapists who use arts therapy in conjunction with other specialties, such as psychiatry and psychology, may earn considerably more. Depending on their education, training, and specialty, psychologists earned between $19,500 and $62,120 in 1997, and creative arts therapists who complete their education in psychology can expect a salary in that range.

Work Environment

Most creative arts therapists work a typical 40-hour, five-day workweek; at times, however, they may have to work extra hours. The number of patients under a therapist's care depends on the specific employment setting. Although many therapists work in hospitals, they may also be employed in such facilities as clinics, rehabilitation centers, children's homes, schools, and nursing homes. Some therapists maintain service contracts with several facilities. For instance, a therapist might work two days a week at a hospital, one day at a nursing home, and the rest of the week at a rehabilitation center.

Most buildings are pleasant, comfortable, and clean places in which to work. Experienced creative arts therapists might choose to be self-employed, working with patients in their own studios. In such a case, the therapist might work more irregular hours to accommodate patient schedules. Other therapists might maintain a combination of service contract work with one or more facilities in addition to a private caseload of clients referred to them by other health care professionals. Whether therapists work on service contracts with various facilities or maintain private practices, they must deal with all of the business and administrative details and worries that go along with being self-employed.

Outlook

The creative arts therapy professions are growing very rapidly, and many new positions are created each year. Although enrollment in college therapy programs is increasing, new graduates are usually able to find jobs. In cases where an individual is unable to find a full-time position, a therapist might obtain service contracts for part-time work at several facilities.

In addition, job openings in facilities such as nursing homes should continue to increase as the elderly population grows over the next few decades. Advances in medical technology and the recent practice of early discharge from hospitals should also create new opportunities in managed care facilities, chronic pain clinics, and cancer care facilities. The demand for therapists of all types should continue to increase as more people become aware of the need to help disabled patients in creative ways. Some drama therapists and psychodramatists are also finding employment opportunities outside of the usual health care field. Such therapists might conduct therapy sessions at corporate sites to enhance the personal effectiveness and growth of employees.

For More Information

For more information about all types of creative arts therapies, contact:

National Coalition of Arts Therapies Associations (NCATA)
2117 L Street, NW, #274
Washington, DC 20037
Tel: 202-678-6787
Web: http://www.ncata.com/

The following organizations can give your more detailed information about your field of interest:

American Art Therapy Association
1202 Allanson Road
Mundelein, IL 60060-3808
Tel: 847-949-6064
Web: http://www.arttherapy.org

American Music Therapy Association
8455 Colesville Road, Suite 1000
Silver Spring, MD 20910
Tel: 301-589-3300
Web: http://www.musictherapy.org/

American Society of Group Psychotherapy and Psychodrama
301 North Harrison Street, Suite 508
Princeton, NJ 08540
Tel: 609-452-1339
Web: http://www.asgpp.org/

National Association for Drama Therapy
5505 Connecticut Avenue, NW, #280
Washington, DC 20015
Tel: 202-966-7409
Web: http://www.nadt.org

National Association for Poetry Therapy (NAPT)
5505 Connecticut Avenue, NW, #280
Washington, DC 20015
Tel: 202-966-2536
Web: http://www.poetrytherapy.org

Ergonomists

School Subjects
Health
Mathematics
Physical education

Personal Skills
Helping/teaching
Mechanical/manipulative

Minimum Education Level
Master's degree

Salary Range
$30,000 to $42,000 to $80,000

Certification or Licensing
Voluntary

Outlook
Faster than the average

Overview

Ergonomists help business, industry, government, and academic institutions use technology responsibly by considering human capabilities and limitations in the workplace. Their goal is to increase human productivity, comfort, safety, and health, and to decrease injury and illness by designing human-centered equipment, furniture, work methods, and techniques. "Ergonomists integrate or combine knowledge derived from the various human sciences to match jobs, systems, products, and environments to the physical and mental abilities and limitations of people," according to the International Ergonomics Association and the Board of Certification in Professional Ergonomics. Ergonomists are also known as *human factors engineers* or *human factors specialists*.

History

"Ergonomics" comes from the Greek word *ergon,* meaning "work." The study of people at work began about 100 years ago as employers and employees began to realize that job productivity was tied to job satisfaction and the nature of the work environment. The concerns of many of the early ergonomists centered around increasing industrial production while maintaining safety on the job. They began to design machines and other equipment that improved production and also reduced the number of job-related accidents. As it became clear that improved working conditions increased productivity and safety and improved workers' morale, ergonomists began investigating other physical and psychological factors that influenced people at work.

Today, with the world of work constantly changing and workplaces using computers and other forms of automation, there is a need for professionals to help adapt the workplace to these changes. About 40 percent of the labor force—or more than 40 million people—now work at computer keyboards and have growing concerns about repetitive strain injuries. According to the National Council on Compensation Insurance Inc., workers' compensation claims related to repetitive strain are up 770 percent from ten years ago. As a result, most major insurance carriers today have ergonomics departments. The ergonomist can help businesses develop methods that will more humanely adapt the workplace to technological changes and also prepare the workplace for the different types of jobs and other changes that are sure to come.

The Job

Ergonomists are concerned with the relationship between people and work, studying and dealing with the limitations and possibilities of the human body. They deal with organizational structure, worker productivity, and job satisfaction. Ergonomists are important consultants on many levels: they help employees work in safer environments, they allow employers to achieve higher levels of productivity, and they educate workers and adapt environments to the task to decrease the number of work-related illnesses and injuries.

Ergonomists work to make sure people can perform their work in the safest manner possible. To be ergonomically sound, a task should allow for three basic principles: it should be able to be completed in several different and safe manners, the largest appropriate muscle groups should be utilized, and joints should be at approximately the middle of their range of movement.

This first principle implies that a task shouldn't be so repetitive that the worker is limited to only one set of movements to complete it. Over time, repetitive actions can lead to muscle and joint trauma. Ergonomists help people avoid repetitive strain injuries. For instance, ergonomists often are called to an assembly line to study the workers' motions. They may suggest different ways for the employees to complete their tasks while still being safe and efficient.

The second principle of ergonomics has to do with muscle work. Larger muscle groups are often better suited to a task than smaller ones. For instance, when lifting a heavy box from the ground, many people automatically bend at the waist and lift the box using the strength in their arms. But this can lead to muscle strain in the arms and the back. A better approach might be to bend at the knees, grip the box to the chest, and lift up slowly, using leg power. By utilizing the longer, stronger leg muscles to lift items, you can reduce your risk of injury. In the workplace, an ergonomist would study how much weight employees have to lift during the day, and perhaps suggest alternate ways to use their bodies or distribute the weight onto different muscle groups.

Finally, proper ergonomic form requires joints to be as close to the middle of their range as possible, which means that you shouldn't hyper- or hypo-extend your arms or legs. Joints perform best when they aren't too straight and aren't too bent. An ergonomist might be called on to help an employee who works at a computer terminal all day. The ergonomist might watch the person at work for a little while, and then determine that the worker's arm and shoulder pain may be caused by the mouse and keyboard placement. If the worker has to extend his arm fully to reach the mouse, he locks his elbow and moves his arm at an unnatural—and uncomfortable—angle.

Guided by these basic principles of ergonomics, ergonomists work with ideas, processes, and people to help make the workplace safer and more comfortable. An ergonomist who deals primarily in design works to create machines and other materials that are both usable and comfortable to the user. This may include physiological research on how certain types of work-related injuries—such as carpal tunnel syndrome—occur. These professionals study mathematics and physics, in conjunction with the human form, in order to gain a better understanding of how people can avoid performing unsafe and repetitive motions that lead to injury.

Other ergonomists adopt a more hands on approach by going out in the field to study a workplace and ascertain the needs of particular employees in specific work situations. Their clients may be as varied as secretaries working in front of the computer, factory workers installing headlights in new automobiles, and travel agents working with telephones propped on their shoulders all day. These ergonomists may study assembly-line procedures and suggest changes to reduce monotony and make it easier for workers to load or unload materials, thereby obtaining optimum efficiency in terms of human capabilities. They may also investigate environmental factors such as lighting and room temperature, which might influence workers' behavior and productivity. In an office setting, an ergonomist is likely to make suggestions about keyboard placement and monitor height to help alleviate injuries. Rearrangement of furniture is often one of the easiest ways to make a workplace safer and more comfortable.

Ergonomists usually work as part of a team, with different specialists focusing on a particular aspect of the work environment. For example, one ergonomist may deal with the safety aspects of machinery, and another may specialize in environmental issues, such as the volume of noise and the layout of the surroundings. After analyzing relevant data and observing how workers interact in the work environment, ergonomists submit a written report of their findings and make recommendations to company executives or representatives for changes or adaptations in the workplace. Their suggestions might be as simple as moving a desk closer to the window to allow for more natural light or installing task lighting to reduce eye strain. They may make proposals for new machinery or suggest a revised design for machinery already in place. They may also suggest environmental changes, like painting walls or soundproofing a noisy work area, so employees can better enjoy the work environment.

Ergonomists may focus on something as large as redesigning the computer terminals for a large multinational corporation, or they may focus on designing more comfortable chairs or easier-to-use telephones at a local family-owned business. Ergonomists may work as consultants for government agencies and manufacturing companies or engage in research at colleges or universities. Often, an ergonomist will specialize in one particular system or application.

Ergonomists are concerned, too, with the social work environment. They are involved with personnel training and development as well as with the interaction between people and machines. Ergonomists may, for example, plan various kinds of tests that will help screen applicants for employment with the firms. They assist engineers and technicians in designing systems that require people and machines to interact. Ergonomists may also develop aids for training people to use those systems.

Requirements

High School

High school is not too early to begin preparing for a career in ergonomics. You should follow a broad college-preparatory curriculum with a concentration in the sciences. Courses in the life and physical sciences—biology, anatomy, health, physics—will be particularly helpful, as will classes in research methods, writing and speech, mathematics, and computer science. Business courses will also help you learn more about the business world and the opportunities available for ergonomists. Any classes that broaden your knowledge of people and how they work and sharpen your skills in communication will be very important. Knowledge of modern foreign languages may also increase opportunities as global, multicultural economies are developing rapidly.

Postsecondary Training

Ergonomists need solid skills in three basic areas: business administration, science and technology, and communications. A career in ergonomics begins with an undergraduate degree in one of the behavioral, biomedical, health, social, or computer sciences or engineering. Potential ergonomists take whichever courses are needed to complete a degree in their chosen field. Most science-based degrees require courses in anatomy, psychology, physiology, statistics, mathematics, and education. If a concentration in ergonomics is available at your college or university, you might take additional courses such as Systems Theory/Operations Research; Demographics, Biomechanics, Kinesiology; Psychology of Learning; Work Analysis and Measurement; Safety and Health Analysis Techniques; Design Methodologies; and Training and Instruction Systems.

Additional courses in business, writing, and communications will help you learn how to communicate your ideas and suggestions to the people with whom you will be working. Again, knowledge of foreign languages will allow you to work more globally.

Most ergonomists also earn a master's degree in industrial engineering or psychology, along with a concentration in ergonomics/human factors. A doctoral degree is an advantage for those who want to pursue research and teaching at the university level or for those who want to develop specialized methodologies for ergonomics in advanced technologies.

Certification or Licensing

Although certification is not mandatory, industry is increasingly recognizing board certification in ergonomics as a standard of professional achievement and skill, and it is recommended that ergonomists earn their credentials to be eligible for the most prime positions. Because ergonomics is a rapidly evolving career field and tied to advances in scientific knowledge and technology, it is especially important to keep up-to-date on the latest developments. To keep current, many ergonomists belong to professional organizations, such as the Human Factors and Ergonomics Society or the Ergonomics and Work Measurement Division of the Institute of Industrial Engineers. Addresses for several such organizations are listed at the end of this article. Ergonomists who work for the federal government may need to pass a civil service examination.

Other Requirements

If you are interested in becoming an ergonomist, you should be able to understand the relationships between actions and their results. An analytic mind is essential, and most ergonomists have good problem-solving skills. If you are interested in the research and design side of ergonomics, you should have good research skills and be able to apply research techniques to practical application. If you prefer to work directly with clients, you should enjoy working with people and be able to illustrate proper ergonomic techniques to them. Finally, empathy is an important trait, since many ergonomists are called on site after an accident or injury has already happened. The ergonomist should be able to investigate the mishap and make recommendations on how to avoid a recurrence and ensure the safety and comfort of the workers.

Exploring

Only those with the required educational credentials can get hands-on experience, so the most practical way to explore career opportunities is to talk with those already working in the field. A great deal of career information can also be found in professional journals. Students may also want to check out some online sources. Many organizations offer electronic newsgroups for people in the industry to discuss news and information about the field. You may wish to subscribe to such a newsgroup or consult Web sites that focus on ergonomics.

After researching the field of ergonomics through published and electronic sources, you may consider trying your hand at setting up an ergonomically sound work area. If you have a computer, you could make sure that the monitor distance, mouse and keyboard placement, and chair height are in accord with accepted ergonomic standards. At school, you might also make sure your desk and locker are put to proper ergonomic use. Place heavy books at the bottom of your locker and bend at the knees to lift them and carry your backpack close to your body with both straps over your shoulders.

Finally, learn to listen to your own body for signs of ergonomic distress. Do your thumbs cramp up after a few hours of video games? That could be an early sign of repetitive stress syndrome and could lead to more serious problems. Before you move on to the next level in *Crash Bandicoot,* press "pause" and stretch out your hands to get the blood flowing again. Does your back hurt after a long day at school? Try to make a conscious effort to sit up straight, with your back straight and lower back flush against the chair. Do your eyeballs get blurry from reading too much? Put down the *Tiger Beat* magazine, put on some good sneakers, and go for a walk.

Employers

Ergonomists are employed by various organizations: hospitals, factories, communications industries, and other businesses. They may be part of the regular staff at a large corporation, or they may work on an as-needed, or contractual, basis. Many ergonomists work as consultants for one or many companies. Ergonomists may practice in tandem with physical therapists, sports medicine practitioners, chiropractors, kinesiologists, and physicians. Those who work in research and design may work with engineers, architects, interior decorators, contractors, and builders.

Because ergonomics is a somewhat new occupation, most positions available will be in larger, more urban areas. Since the government also hires ergonomists to work in various organizations, one of the largest concentrations of ergonomists is in Washington, DC. The field is evolving at a rapid pace, and skilled ergonomists will be able to forge their own way in the profession.

Starting Out

Since it's a relatively new profession, people looking to enter the ergonomic field will have many ways to get started. Some will complete their undergraduate and graduate degrees prior to getting a job in the profession. Others may prefer to work full time while earning their credentials part time. Still others may work on the fringes of ergonomics before earning certification. These folks may have expertise in other areas, such as sports medicine, architecture, or engineering. Often, an interest in preventing injuries rather than treating them leads many people from the medical field to a career in ergonomics. In any case, most certification programs require some professional experience in the field prior to certification.

Your first job in ergonomics can let you shape your own career. If you are interested in using ergonomics in a sport setting, for instance, you could try getting a job as a consultant to a minor league sports team in your community. If you think you would prefer working in a more businesslike environment, you should get a job with an established ergonomic service. Professional organizations usually have job listings and career assistance, and many colleges and universities offer career guidance to their graduates. If you plan on using ergonomics training for your own consultation business, it's often a good idea to do an internship or assistantship with an established ergonomist or group of ergonomists in order to practice your skills and build a client base.

Advancement

Because ergonomics is still rapidly evolving, advancement opportunities are considered good for the near future. There are not that many people involved in the field and, therefore, there are many opportunities for qualified individuals, especially those who have a special area of expertise. Many ergonomists develop skills at a first job and then either use that experience to find higher paid work at a different company or to get increased responsibility in their current position.

Qualified ergonomists often are promoted to management positions, with an accompanying increase in earnings and responsibility. They can also start their own consulting firms or branch off into teaching or research. Those in government work may choose to move to the private sector, where salaries are higher. But others may opt for the security and job responsibilities of a government position.

Earnings

Earnings depend on the individual's education, experience, and type of work sought. Beginning ergonomists may earn anywhere from $30,000 to $60,000 per year; those with a doctorate earn more. Experienced ergonomists often earn $70,000 to $80,000 a year, especially those who work in private industry. Those with a doctorate tend to earn more than those with a master's degree. Full-time employees usually receive health insurance, vacation, and other benefits.

Ergonomists who work as consultants usually get paid a negotiated fee, with rates ranging from $60 to $200 per hour, depending on their skill and reputation, the area of the country where they work, and the industry. These consultants have more control over their working hours, but usually do not receive health insurance or other benefits. Many ergonomists may hold a full-time position and then consult or teach part time.

Work Environment

Ergonomists encounter various working conditions, depending on specific duties and responsibilities. An ergonomist may work in a typical office environment, with computer and data processing equipment close at hand. The ergonomist may also work in a factory, investigating production problems. Usually, ergonomists do both: they work in an office setting and make frequent visits to a factory or other location to work out particular production issues. Although the majority of the work is not strenuous, ergonomists may occasionally assemble or revamp machinery or work processes. They also spend much of their time explaining procedures and techniques to their clients.

Ergonomists often work as part of a team, but they may also work on an individual research project, spending much time alone, doing research at the library or online, or working out a production schedule on the computer. They usually work a 40-hour week, although overtime and odd hours are not uncommon, especially if a particular project is on deadline or there are urgent safety issues at hand. There may be occasional weekend and evening work, depending on the industry and project. Those involved with research or teaching may only work ten months a year, although many of these ergonomists work as consultants when not employed full time.

Outlook

As the work environment becomes more complex and workers expect more from their jobs (and employers expect more from their workers), the opportunities for ergonomists continue to grow. This trend is expected to continue well into the twenty-first century. The occupation should be somewhat insulated from changes in the economy. If the economy grows, more companies will need to adapt workplaces to increase production capabilities. If the economy slows down, many companies will need to cut costs and improve productivity. The skilled ergonomist can make both scenarios profitable for the business and the individual employees.

The majority of ergonomists now work for large manufacturing firms, and this should continue into the future. As ergonomics becomes more established, driving down costs, smaller firms will be better able to use ergonomists for consultation. Computer companies and others that use automated systems will need ergonomists to help them develop effective and stimulating work environments. The government also hires experts who can design safe and productive work environments. Colleges, universities, and other research facilities need ergonomists to interpret data and supply new ideas for productive work environments. Some ergonomists will be freelance consultants.

For More Information

For full details about the certification process for ergonomists, contact:

Board of Certification in Professional Ergonomics
PO Box 2811
Bellingham, WA 98227-2811
Tel: 360-671-7601
Web: http://www.bcpe.org

Human Factors and Ergonomics Society
PO Box 1369
Santa Monica, CA 90406
Tel: 310-394-1811
Web: http://www.hfes.org/

Herbalists

School Subjects
Biology
Chemistry
Earth science

Personal Skills
Helping/teaching
Technical/scientific

Work Environment
Primarily indoors
Primarily one location

Minimum Education Level
Associate's degree

Salary Range
$13,000 to $70,000 to $200,000

Certification or Licensing
Required by certain states

Outlook
Faster than the average

Overview

Herbalists are health care professionals who practice healing through the use of herbs. The same term applies to individuals who grow and collect herbs. *Herbs* are plants or plant parts—roots, bark, leaves, flowers, or berries—that are used for their aromatic, savory, or medicinal qualities. Herbs, which are sometimes called *botanicals* are now the fastest growing category in drugstores because of the steadily increasing interest in herbal preparations.

The field of herbalism is expanding and changing rapidly. Professional herbalists work in a variety of places. Some are primary health care providers; some work as consultants in health care settings. Others work in health food stores or are employed by herbalists. A few grow or harvest herbs. Some manufacture or market herbs and herbal products. Still others work in companies overseeing the quality control of raw materials and/or overseeing product education and research. In 1998, there were roughly 15,000 professional herbalists in the United States.

History

Long before recorded history, early humans undoubtedly used plants and plant products not only for food but also for medicine. Between 8000 and 5000 BC, early people are known to have gathered or cultivated more than 200 plants. A number of those plants had medicinal qualities.

The folk medicine traditions of all cultures include the use of plants and plant products. Knowledge of herbs and herbal remedies has been handed down from generation to generation and from culture to culture. Ancient cultures—such as the Babylonian, Chinese, Egyptian, and Syrian—developed detailed *pharmacopoeias* (books describing medical preparations) that included many commonly used herbs.

In the Orient, the Chinese developed a complete system of herbal medicine called *Chinese herbology.* The earliest work, the Yellow Emperor's *Classic of Internal Medicine* (*Huang Di Nei Ching*) was recorded around 2,300 years ago. Like other aspects of traditional Chinese medicine, Chinese herbology is based upon the principle of restoring balance to the individual's vital energy, which is called *qi* (or *chi,* both pronounced "chee"). Chinese herbology remains a distinct form of herbalism today.

In the West, the Egyptians developed and recorded herbal medicinal systems. The *Kahun Medical Papyrus* dates back to 1900 BC. Hippocrates and other early Greek physicians used herbs and other natural remedies to heal their patients. Some of their knowledge was based on early Egyptian herbal medicine. The work of the early Egyptian and Greek healers evolved into what is now considered Western herbalism.

European settlers brought their herbs and herbal remedies with them to this country. They also brought *herbals*—books on herbal medicine. The settlers learned about the herbs of the New World from the Native Americans and through their own observations. In 1751, John Bartram, one of the most respected botanists of the colonial era, published a list of indigenous North American plants and their uses.

Even into the early 20th century, much of the pharmacopoeia of conventional medical practitioners was based on the herbal lore of native peoples. Many of the drugs we commonly use today are of herbal origin. It is estimated that 75 percent of modern drugs were originally derived from plants and that about 20 percent still are. With the rise of modern medicine, herbal and other natural remedies fell out of popularity for a time.

With the immense popular interest in alternative medicine in the last three decades of the 20th century, interest in and demand for herbal products has skyrocketed. In Europe (especially England, Germany, and Switzerland), botanicals have long been considered important complements to conventional drugs. Herbal remedies are also more generally accepted and used in Australia, Japan, India, China, and some African countries. The United States is just beginning to catch up with the rest of the world in recognizing the value of the medicinal use of herbs.

Throughout the history of humanity, men and women have practiced herbalism on a daily basis. The World Health Organization (WHO), which is the medical branch of the United Nations, estimates that 80 percent of the world's population presently utilizes traditional healing practices that include herbal medicine in some way in primary health care.

The Job

There are several kinds of herbalists in the United States. Their job descriptions vary widely depending upon the area of the herbal industry in which they work. According to Roy Upton, Vice-President of the American Herbalists Guild, herbalists who want to practice primarily as health care professionals have two basic options. They can become primary health care providers or they can work as allied health professionals, that is, more as consultants than as practitioners. In the United States at this time, there are two officially recognized forms of training for herbalists: Oriental medicine and naturopathy.

Oriental medicine practitioners are trained in Chinese herbology. They study approximately 300 herbs and 125 herbal formulas, including their actions, indications, contraindications, side effects, and standard formulas. *Chinese herbalists* practice herbal science according to the philosophy and principals of Oriental medicine. First, they perform a careful evaluation and diagnosis of the client's situation. Next, they consider all of the person's characteristics and symptoms to determine what is out of balance in the person's qi. Oriental medicine practitioners believe that the body's energy flows along specific channels—called meridians—in the body. Each meridian relates to a particular physiological system and internal organ. When qi is unbalanced, or when its flow along the channels is blocked or disrupted, disease, pain, and other physical and emotional conditions result. Finally, Chinese herbalists select the proper herb or combination of herbs to use in a strategy for restoring balance to the individual's qi. Chinese herbalists sometimes develop special herbal formulas based upon their diagnosis of the unique combination of the individual's characteristics, symptoms, and primary complaints.

Naturopaths (pronounced "nature-o-paths") are trained for many years in a distinct system of health care called naturopathy. They use a variety of natural approaches to health and healing, including herbal medicine. Like Chinese herbalists, naturopaths recognize the integrity of the whole person, and they consider all of the patient's characteristics and symptoms in planning a course of treatment. If they select an herbal remedy as the appropriate approach, they may use Chinese herbs or Western herbs. Naturopathic physicians study approximately 100 herbs. Unlike Chinese herbalists, they do not base their choice of herbs on the philosophy and principles of Oriental medicine. Compared to Chinese herbalists, naturopaths learn few standard herbal formulas, and they do not usually develop their own formulas. Naturopaths take a more Western approach to the use of herbal medicine, and they are more likely to prescribe a particular herbal medicine based upon a particular diagnosis.

Many *professional herbalists* have studied herbalism extensively but are not certified as Oriental medicine practitioners or licensed as naturopathic physicians. Some of them use their knowledge of herbal therapeutics to help their clients improve their health and their lives. They usually describe their services very carefully in order to avoid being charged with practicing medicine without a license. According to Mr. Upton, "In rare instances, herbalists have been integrated into managed care programs as herbalist consultants, much as registered dieticians have been integrated into the fabric of the health care delivery system. Their scope of practice is limited."

With the surge of interest in alternative health care and natural approaches to medicine, the demand for botanicals increased dramatically during the 1990s. As a result, a growing number of herbalists work in health food stores, drugstores, and other retail stores. There they decide which botanicals to order, monitor the stock, and help customers understand the myriad of products available.

A few herbalists become *wildcrafters*—individuals who collect herbs that grow naturally outdoors. They may need to have permission or permits to take herbs from particular areas. They follow very detailed guidelines about which herbs to harvest—and exactly when and how to collect them. Wildcrafters need to be trained to know which species are sensitive or endangered and how to avoid harming them.

Some herbalists grow herbs for sale. They must know exactly the right conditions for growing herbs, how to select good plants, and how to harvest, store, and ship them properly.

Other herbalists work in the manufacture and distribution of botanicals. Their duties include quality control, literature review, and development of technical, educational, and promotional materials for products. They give educational seminars for health professionals, retailers, and consumers. They may also be called upon to provide technical support to consumers and health professionals and to conduct market analyses.

Herbalists also become teachers. Those who are certified in Oriental medicine or licensed as naturopathic physicians work in colleges and universities that teach the approaches in which they are trained. A few professional herbalists run their own schools. They offer a variety of programs, and some offer certificates of completion. Some also become writers.

Many who work in the various areas of herbalism run their own businesses. Like all business owners, they recruit, hire, and train staff. To be successful, they must maintain detailed records about their businesses.

Requirements

High School

To prepare yourself for a career as an herbalist, take classes in agriculture, botany, ecology, and horticulture so you can learn about plants and how they are grown. Biology, chemistry, and physics will help prepare you to study the properties of herbs and their therapeutic uses. If you want to become a health care practitioner, you'll be taking a lot of medical courses in college, so premed classes will be especially helpful. Nearly all health care professions involve interacting with people. Classes in psychology, English, debate, and drama can help you develop good communication skills. If you become an herbalist, business and computer skills will be important because you are likely to have your own business.

Postsecondary Training

If Chinese herbology will be your path toward a career as an herbalist, you will study six to eight years after high school. Oriental medicine schools offer specialties in Chinese herbology. Most are master's level programs. For admission, you need two years of undergraduate study or a bachelor's degree in a related field, such as science, nursing, or premed. Most programs provide a thorough education in Chinese herbology, other aspects of traditional Oriental medicine, and Western sciences.

More than 40 Oriental medicine schools in the United States offer courses in Chinese herbology. Choosing a school can be complex. State requirements to practice Oriental medicine and Chinese herbology vary, so be sure the school you choose will prepare you to practice in your state. The Oriental medicine associations listed at the end of this article have information on school programs and obtaining financial assistance.

If your path toward becoming an herbalist will have a more Western flavor, you will study naturopathic medicine. Becoming a naturopathic physician requires eight years of study after high school. First, you complete a premed undergraduate program including courses in herbal sciences, chemistry, other basic medical sciences, nutrition, and psychology.

The naturopathic doctoral degree is a four-year program. It includes courses in botanical medicine and other basic medical sciences. You will also take courses in nutrition, homeopathy, and minor surgery. In addition to course instruction, you will receive extensive clinical training. When you finish, you will have a Doctor of Naturopathic Medicine degree (ND or sometimes NMD).

Contact the accredited naturopathic colleges as early as possible to ensure that you complete the prerequisite courses. Accredited schools offer the Doctor of Naturopathic Medicine degree. Schools without accreditation offer correspondence courses and may offer certificates. Only a degree from an accredited school will prepare you to become a licensed naturopath. The professional naturopathic associations listed at the end of this article can help you learn about accredited schools and their requirements.

At this time, no colleges or universities offer specific programs in herbalism for those who are interested in becoming professional herbalists without following either of the career paths detailed above. Individually run herbal schools generally accept those who have a genuine interest in the field. Some offer certificates of completion, but there is no established career path to follow.

Certification or Licensing

Certification indicates that an individual meets the standards established by a professional organization. Licensing is a requirement established by a government body that grants individuals the right to practice within the state.

For Chinese herbalists, the National Certification Commission for Acupuncture and Oriental Medicine (NCCAOM) provides certification and promotes nationally recognized standards for Chinese herbology and Oriental medicine. In order to qualify to take the NCCAOM exam, you must meet educational and/or practice requirements.

Licensing requirements for Oriental medicine practitioners vary widely from state to state, and they are changing rapidly. Nearly 40 states license Oriental medicine practitioners. The national Oriental medicine organizations are great sources for the most up-to-date information about certification and licensing requirements.

For herbalists who are naturopaths, to practice medicine as a naturopathic physician, you must be licensed in the state in which you practice. Licensing is available in 12 states: Alaska, Arizona, Connecticut, Florida, Hawaii, Maine, Montana, New Hampshire, Oregon, Utah, Vermont, and Washington. To become licensed, all 12 states require that you pass the Naturopathic Physicians Licensing Exam (NPLEX), a standardized test for all naturopathic physicians in North America.

Naturopaths who practice in unlicensed states are not allowed to practice as physicians, but they can still use their skills and knowledge to help people improve their lives.

The American Herbalists Guild (AHG) offers peer review for professional herbalists who specialize in the medicinal use of plants. Members voluntarily submit to a peer-review process that is designed to promote and maintain excellence in herbalism. They also adhere to a code of ethics developed by the AHG. There is no other recognized certification or licensing for professional herbalists at this time.

Other Requirements

To be a successful herbalist, you need a profound respect for and enjoyment of nature. Like other health care practitioners, herbalists often work with people who may be ill or in pain. You need compassion and understanding for your clients and a strong desire to help them improve their lives. Good listening skills and a reassuring manner are helpful. Strong intuition, careful observation, and good mystery-solving skills are also valuable. Idealism, the courage of your convictions, and willingness to stand up for your beliefs are essential. Herbalism and other alternative health care approaches have become much more respected and accepted in recent years, but they are still misunderstood by many people.

Exploring

Numerous opportunities to learn about the field of herbalism are available. Go to health food stores and Chinese herb shops. Look through the books and periodicals they offer. Talk to the people who run the shops—chances are they are herbalists. Ask them about their field and how they like it. Perhaps you can get a part-time job there to learn more.

Join a local horticulture society. Plant a garden or grow plants in containers or a window garden. The professional associations listed at the end of this chapter have many programs and workshops that are available to everyone. Some have student memberships.

The Internet has a wealth of information. Some Web sites have chat groups; others have searchable herbal databases. If you find you are seriously interested, consider taking a seminar or a correspondence course from one of the privately run herbal schools.

Employers

Most Chinese herbalists and herbalists who are naturopaths operate private practices. Some form or join partnerships with practitioners of other alternative health care modalities. Professionals and clinics in other areas of health care, such as chiropractors, osteopaths, and M.D.s, may employ herbalists as consultants. As Oriental medicine and naturopathy are becoming more accepted, there are growing opportunities with universities and within government agencies for research into herbal medicine.

Major employers of professional herbalists are dietary supplement manufacturers, health food retailers, pharmaceutical companies, and educational organizations. The largest concentration of manufacturers is in California. Other employers can be found throughout the country. Herbalists who work as consultants, wildcrafters, manufacturers, educators, and writers are usually self-employed.

Starting Out

Herbalists who study naturopathy and Chinese herbology frequently get help from their schools for initial placement. When starting out, some herbalists find jobs in clinics with doctors or chiropractors or in wellness centers. This gives them a chance to start practicing in a setting where they can work with and learn from others. Some begin working with more experienced practitioners and later go into private practice. Both Chinese herbalists and naturopaths frequently work in private practice.

When you start out as a Chinese herbal therapist or as a naturopath, one of the most important considerations is having the proper certification and licensing for your geographical area. This is essential because the requirements for the professions, for each state, and for the nation are changing so rapidly.

For other herbalists, there are no formal career pathways. Networking is a major way to make the connections that lead to jobs. You can get to know people in the herbal community through the Internet, by joining associations, and by attending meetings.

For a career in retailing, identify health food stores and other retailers that offer herbal products, and talk to the store manager. If you are interested in the manufacturing and distribution areas, attend trade shows and send your resume to manufacturers. As in many other fields, finding a mentor can be extremely helpful.

Advancement

Because most naturopaths and Chinese herbalists work in private or group practice, advancement frequently depends on their dedication to building up a client base. As an herbalist in private practice, you will need a general sense of how to run a successful business. You will need to promote your practice within the community and develop a network of contacts with conventional medical doctors or other alternative practitioners who may refer clients to you.

Other herbalists advance through increasing their knowledge of the part of the industry in which they work. An individual who works in retail could become the manager of the department or store. An herb grower or wildcrafter might employ others and expand the business. Those in manufacturing and distribution may have opportunities for foreign travel. Some advance by starting their own businesses.

Herbalists who become distinguished in their fields can become self-employed and consult, write, or teach. With the growing government interest in research into natural health care, more naturopathic physicians and Chinese herbalists will find opportunities for advancement as researchers.

Earnings

Earnings of course vary according to an herbalist's specialty. For self-employed herbalists, income is usually closely related to the number of hours worked and the rates charged. Starting pay for a private Oriental medicine practitioner specializing in Chinese herbology may be $13,000 to $20,000 until the practice builds. Rates increase with experience. Clinics might offer $15,000 to $20,000 to start. An average income for full-time Oriental medicine practitioners is $35,000 to $50,000. A very experienced Oriental medicine practitioner with a well-established practice can sometimes net $200,000 or more.

A beginning naturopath earns around $35,000 a year. After some years of practice, NDs generally average $80,000 to $100,000 per year. Though a well-established naturopath can potentially make up to $200,000 a year, most earn much less.

In manufacturing and retail positions, beginning earnings range from $35,000 to $40,000. Mid-level wages are generally from $40,000 to $70,000, and highly skilled, experienced individuals earn from $70,000 to $200,000. Like other self-employed individuals, herbalists in private practice must provide their own insurance, vacation, and retirement benefits. Herbalists who are employed in industry, at universities, or as researchers generally receive some benefits, such as health insurance, sick pay and vacation pay, and contributions to retirement funds.

Work Environment

Herbalists who specialize in Oriental herbal medicine or naturopathy usually work indoors in clean, quiet, comfortable offices. Since most are in private practice, they define their own surroundings. Private practitioners set their own hours, but many work some evenings and weekends to accommodate their patients' schedules. They usually work without supervision and must have a lot of self-discipline.

For herbalists who work in clinics, research settings, and universities, the surroundings vary. Wherever they work, health care practitioners need clean, quiet offices. In these larger settings, herbalists must be good team players. They may also need to work well under supervision.

Herbalists who are employed in retail, manufacture, or distribution may find themselves in a variety of settings, however most of their work is indoors. Their jobs may involve travel within the United States or even abroad. They must work well in a group environment, enjoy working with people, and work well under pressure. Wildcrafters and herb growers spend time both indoors and outdoors. They work with plants, soil, and equipment. They may work alone or with others.

Outlook

With the American public's rapidly increasing interest in alternative health care and natural health remedies, herbalists will be in demand in the early 21st century. Mainstream magazines and newspapers, television, and the Internet are full of articles and advertisements telling of the virtues and successes of herbal therapies.

Sales of herbal supplements have increased dramatically since 1993. Some respected sources report increases in herb sales as high as 35 percent in the mass market and as high as 20 percent for the industry as a whole. Roy Upton of the American Herbalists Guild projects that the employment outlook will be excellent for those who pursue an herbal education with a strong science background, or the reverse.

Both naturopathic physicians and Oriental medicine practitioners are expected to be in demand as well, so herbalists trained in those fields should have good employment opportunities. Demands for naturopaths and all aspects of Oriental medicine are growing rapidly due to increasing public awareness and acceptance. Interest from the mainstream medical community, recent advances in research, and favorable changes in government policy are strong indicators that these areas will continue to expand. In both fields, the demand for these alternative health care professionals exceeds the number available.

For More Information

A national professional association for information about naturopathic medicine, accredited schools, and state licensing status:

American Association of Naturopathic Physicians
601 Valley Street, Suite 105
Seattle, WA 98109
Tel: 206-298-0126
Web: http://www.naturopathic.org

A national education association dedicated to educating the public about beneficial herbs and plants and to promoting safe use of medicinal plants:

American Botanical Council (ABC)
PO Box 144345
Austin, TX 78714-4345
Tel: 512-926-4900
Web: http:/www.herbalgram.org

A national educational organization that promotes excellence in herbalism and provides peer review for professional herbalists:

American Herbalists Guild
PO Box 70
Roosevelt, UT 84066
Tel: 435-722-8434
Web: http://www.healthy.net/pan/pa/Herbalmedicine/ahg/index.html

The national trade association that represents the herbal and herbal products industry:

American Herbal Products Association
8484 Georgia Avenue, Suite 370
Silver Spring, MD 20910
Tel: 301-588-1171
Web: http://www.healthy.net/pan/trade/ahpa/index.html

A research and educational organization that provides information on herbs to the public and to professionals:

Herb Research Foundation
1007 Pearl Street, Suite 200
Boulder, CO 80302
Tel: 303-449-2265
Web: http://www.herbs.org

An organization that is open to anyone interested in herbs and is dedicated to promoting the use and delight of herbs:

Herb Society of America
9019 Kirtland Chardon Road
Kirtland, OH 44094
Tel: 440-256-0514
Web: http://www.herbsociety.org

Holistic Dentists

	School Subjects
Biology Business Chemistry	
	Personal Skills
Technical/scientific Mechanical/manipulative	
	Work Environment
Primarily indoors Primarily one location	
	Minimum Education Level
Medical degree	
	Salary Range
$80,000 to $120,000 to $175,000	
	Certification or Licensing
Required by all states	
	Outlook
About as fast as the average	

Overview

Holistic dentists are health care professionals who use an approach to the practice of dentistry that considers the patient as a whole person—including mind, body, and spirit. They consider the potential effects any dental procedure may have on the entire individual.

Holistic dentists represent a small but steadily growing number of dentists in the United States. An increasing number of dentists incorporate holistic approaches into their practices without necessarily declaring themselves to be holistic dentists. At this time, the American Dental Association (ADA) does not recognize holistic dentistry as a specialty. Like most other dentists, the majority of holistic dentists work in private practice.

History

As long as 5,000 years ago, healing traditions of India, China, and other ancient cultures promoted living a healthy life in harmony with nature—a concept that is central to a holistic approach to dentistry. The earliest texts of ancient civilizations, such as China, India, and Egypt, detail treatments for toothache.

Hippocrates, who is sometimes considered to be the father of Western medicine, taught his students to assess the living environment of their patients in order to understand their illnesses. Hippocrates is known to have developed natural dentifrice and mouthwash.

For centuries, healers, surgeons, and even barbers practiced dentistry. It was not until the 16th and 17th centuries that dentistry emerged as a specialty with its own literature.

In 1728, Pierre Fauchard, a French dentist, published the textbook *The Surgeon Dentist*. His writings encouraged a broader education for dentists and elevated dental treatment to a more scientific level. As a result of his work, Fauchard is sometimes considered the father of modern dentistry.

Between 1844 and 1846, Horace Wells and William Morton—both dentists—introduced general anesthesia to medicine. Their efforts (and the efforts of others who tried to find ways to make dental procedures less traumatic for the patient) showed an understanding of the effects dental treatment has on the entire person.

In 1910, two Englishmen, Sir William Hunter and Sir Kenneth Goodby, pointed out that infected teeth could cause infection to spread throughout the entire body.

The modern term "holism" was first used in 1926 by Jan Smuts in his book *Holism and Evolution*. Smuts championed the idea that living things are much more than just the sum of their parts. He challenged modern medical science, which denied the complexity of the human experience by reducing the individual to a collection of body parts and diseases.

During the middle of the 20th century, scientific medical advances focused on germs—outside sources of disease. Being healthy became a matter of overcoming disease, and people looked to modern doctors and dentists to fix their ills. For a time, holistic health concepts fell out of favor in the United States.

However, in the last decades of the 20th century, the general public became increasingly aware that modern medicine did not have all the answers. By the 1970s, "holistic" had become a common term. During the 1980s and 1990s, holistic principles were increasingly incorporated into individual lifestyles and into the practice of medicine and dentistry.

The Job

Holistic dentistry is as much a philosophy as it is a particular set of practices. Holistic dentists consider the ramifications of dental care on the whole person, and they consider the patient to be a partner in the healing process.

In many ways, the primary duties of holistic dentists are very similar to those of other dentists. They examine patients' teeth, diagnose problem areas, fill cavities, treat areas with gum disease, repair broken teeth, and extract teeth when necessary. Some perform corrective surgery to treat gum disease. They administer anesthetics for the relief or prevention of pain during dental procedures, and they prescribe medications. They instruct patients in caring for their teeth—including proper diet, brushing, flossing, and other aspects of preventive maintenance.

The main difference between holistic dentists and more conventional dentists is in their approach to the client/dentist relationship. Holistic dentists consider themselves to be partners with their patients in the process of helping to enhance the health and well being of the whole individual—body, mind, and spirit. They consider the effects that any procedure may have on the entire person, not just on the physical being. They emphasize prevention and their clients' responsibility for taking an active role their own health care.

Some holistic dentists use alternative therapies. They take special care to use aromatherapy in their offices to create an environment in which clients can feel comfortable and at ease. They may also use aromatherapies known for their germicidal properties. Homeopathic remedies may be given to relieve pain or to dissipate the effects of anesthesia more quickly. Holistic dentists use nutritional counseling to encourage their patients to take a more active role in improving their health and wellness. They may refer individuals who have special needs to homeopaths or nutritionists.

Holistic dentists use an interdisciplinary approach to health care to facilitate the body's innate ability to heal itself. They differ widely in the methods they use to accomplish that goal. While many incorporate other alternative therapies into their practices, others do not.

In keeping with their philosophy of considering the effects of a treatment on the entire person, holistic dentists minimize or avoid the use of some common dental procedures that they consider potentially harmful. Once again, they vary greatly in their determinations of what is harmful. Some avoid X rays, mercury-based fillings, and fluoride treatments; others do not.

Holistic dentists range from those who use mostly conventional methods and incorporate a few alternative ideas to those use mostly unconventional approaches. While the methods they choose may vary greatly, their approaches to patients have more in common.

In order to understand the whole person, holistic dentists generally spend much more time with their patients than conventional dentists. They discuss possible courses of treatment and involve their patients in decisions about which procedures and materials to use, and they encourage questions. An initial appointment may take an hour and a half, and a routine appointment usually takes 45 minutes to an hour.

In addition to their regular duties as health care providers, holistic dentists must complete an enormous amount of paperwork. Whether they work in clinics or in private practice, they keep accurate patient records. More and more insurance companies are covering dental services. Holistic dental practitioners must frequently submit records to insurance companies in order to be paid for their services.

According to the American Dental Association, nearly 90 percent of dentists are in private practice. They are responsible for setting up, advertising, promoting, and running their own businesses. They have to recruit, hire, and train staff. They also oversee the purchase and care of dental equipment and supplies. Holistic dentists in private practice may spend a large percentage of their time on business matters.

To maintain their licenses, dentists must take continuing education courses. Holistic dentists usually take many more hours than required to maintain their licenses because they want to maintain the skills they need for this interdisciplinary approach to health care.

Requirements

High School

If you are interested in a career in holistic dentistry, take as many science classes as possible, especially chemistry, biology, and physics. Science classes will help you learn the type of thinking process you need for dentistry, and they will help prepare you for dentistry courses. Art classes can also be helpful because dentists need to have good manual dexterity and excellent judgment of space and shape. Taf Paulson, D.D.S., a holistic dentist in Chicago, says she considers an important part of her work to be "putting little pieces of beautiful sculpture into peoples' mouths to help them be healthier."

Holistic dentists need to communicate well and compassionately with their patients. Psychology, English, speech, and debate can help you sharpen your communication skills. Business, mathematics, and computer courses will help you gain the skills you need to be a successful businessperson.

Postsecondary Training

Dental schools require at least two years of college-level predental education, with emphasis on science. However, most students entering dental school have at least a bachelor's degree. Take as many science courses as possible—especially chemistry.

Since holistic dentistry is not yet taught as a specialty, you have the opportunity to plan your own. During undergraduate school, you will have more freedom to choose your classes, so take advantage of the opportunity. Courses in nutrition, homeopathy, and psychology will give you some of the background you need to develop your own holistic dentistry specialty.

In addition to educational preparation, all dental schools require that you pass the Dental Admissions Test (DAT). In selecting students, the schools consider your DAT score, overall grade point average (GPA), science course GPA, and any recommendations. You will also have a personal interview at the school to you which you apply, which will count in the selection process.

Dental school usually takes four years. During the first two years, you will have classroom instruction and laboratory work. Your courses will include anatomy, biochemistry, microbiology, and physiology and beginning classes in clinical sciences. During the last two years, you will treat patients under the supervision of licensed dentists. When you finish, you will have the degree of Doctor of Dental Surgery (D.D.S.) or Doctor of Dental Medicine (D.M.D.), depending on the school you attend.

Certification or Licensing

Like conventional dentists, holistic dentists must be licensed in all 50 states and the District of Columbia. In most states, in order to take the test, you must graduate from a dental school accredited by the American Dental Association's Commission on Dental Accreditation and pass written and practical examinations. Holistic dentistry is not presently considered a specialty, so only a general license is necessary for holistic dental practitioners.

Other Requirements

To be a successful holistic dentist, you need to enjoy people, have a caring attitude, and have a sincere desire to help others improve their lives. Communication with patients is central to holistic dentistry, so excellent listening and communication skills are important.

Idealism, strong convictions, and high ethical standards are essential. Alternative health care approaches have become more respected within the dental community in recent years, but many dentists still do not accept them. It helps to be a bit of a crusader.

Attention to detail and strong powers of observation are crucial to accurate dental assessment. You also need to be an innovative thinker and good mystery solver. When one approach to a situation doesn't work, you need to be able to quickly think of another. Dentists should have a high degree of manual dexterity. They also need good visual memory and excellent judgment of space and shape.

Most dentists work in private practice, so you will need good business sense and a lot of self-discipline.

Exploring

To find out if a career as a holistic dentist is for you, you can explore the field in a variety of ways. Join science clubs to see if a career in a scientific field really interests you.

Visit your local health food stores and explore the nutrition, homeopathic, herbal, and aromatherapy sections. Talk with the staff. You may find some very knowledgeable, helpful people. Pick up any alternative newspapers and magazines they have.

Contact the professional associations listed at the end of this article for information. The Internet has a wealth of information. Some Web sites have chat groups; others have searchable databases.

Go to a holistic dentist for a dental exam. Experience how the dentist works, and think about whether you would like to practice dentistry this way. Talk with the dentist about the field. Perhaps that person would be willing to hire you for a summer or part-time position or become your mentor.

Employers

The main employers of holistic dentists are other dentists who have similar beliefs about dentistry and have large practices or group practices. A number of holistic dentists become salaried employees of group practices and work as associate dentists. Working for other dentists is usually less expensive initially but also less financially rewarding. A few holistic dentists may work in private and public hospitals, in clinics, or in dental research.

Most holistic dentists practice on their own or with a partner. Working with a partner makes practicing easier because the costs of running an office are shared. Other tasks, such as bookkeeping and record keeping can also be shared. However, according to the 1998-99 *Occupational Outlook Handbook,* nine out of ten dentists are in private practice.

Starting Out

The dental school you attend will have listings for job openings for dentists. Professional dental journals, daily newspapers, and the Internet also have listings.

Networking is always one of the best ways to find employment. Join professional organizations, attend meetings, and get to know people in the field. You never know who might know someone who knows someone who is hiring. By meeting people in the field, you have a better chance of learning which dentists share some of your philosophies about holistic dentistry.

Working in the practice or clinic of another physician who shares your beliefs about the practice of dentistry is one of the best ways to get started as a holistic dentist. It is hard to learn in isolation. When you interview potential employers, learn about their approaches to dentistry. Be sure the setting will help you apply the skills you have learned without compromising what you believe about good dental practices.

Most recent dental graduates go into private practice right away. Some set up a new practice. Dental schools have resources to help you learn how to set up your own practice. Some recent graduates purchase an established practice from a dentist who is retiring or moving.

Advancement

As with many professions, advancement in the holistic dental profession usually means building a larger practice. A holistic dentist who starts out as a salaried employee in a large practice may eventually become a partner in the practice. Dentists also advance their careers by building their clientele and setting up their own group practices. They sometimes buy the practices of retiring practitioners to add to their own.

Specialization is another way to advance. Holistic dentists might specialize in pediatric dentistry or geriatric dentistry. Another avenue for advancement is continuing education. Holistic dentistry requires even more continual learning than conventional dentistry. All dentists are required to take 36 hours of continuing education every two years. Some holistic dentists may take as many as 125 hours per year to keep up on developments in areas such as homeopathy, aromatherapy, or nutrition in addition to conventional dental education.

Earnings

Holistic dentists can generally earn about as much as conventional dentists who work in the same settings. Some holistic dentists may earn less because they spend more time with their patients, so they can see fewer in a day. Some make up the difference by charging more per visit.

According to the American Dental Association, the median net income of dentists in general practice was around $109,000 per year in 1995. Those in private practice earned about $120,000, while those in specialty practices earned about $175,000 a year. In the beginning years of practice, dentists often earn less. Those in mid-career tend to earn more.

Since most holistic dentists are self-employed, they must arrange for their own benefits. Those who work for other dentists or in clinics or research may receive insurance, paid sick days and holidays, and other benefits.

Work Environment

Holistic dentists work in particularly clean, quiet, comfortable offices. Making the office healthful, comfortable, and pleasant is of particular importance to many holistic dentists. Some use air filtration systems and aromatherapy. They may also use distilled water instead of tap water. They choose ergonomically appropriate furniture and work stations.

Most solo practitioners and group practices have an office suite. The suite generally has a reception area. In clinics, several professionals may share this area. Most dentists have a secretary or office staff. Some employ dental assistants and dental hygienists to handle routine services.

Holistic dentists who work in large practices or clinics need to work well in a group environment. They may work under supervision or in a team with other professionals.

Most holistic dentists work four to five days a week. Most work around 40 hours a week, although some put in longer hours. Larger practices and clinics may determine the hours of work, but holistic dentists in private practice can set their own hours. Evening and weekend hours may be scheduled to accommodate patients.

Outlook

The 1998-99 *Occupational Outlook Handbook* (OOH) projects that demand for dental care should increase substantially through the year 2006. The largest segment of the population—the baby boomers—will be likely to need complicated dental work as they advance into middle age. People are living longer, and the elderly are more likely to retain their teeth than earlier generations. That means they will continue to need dental care.

The employment of dentists is not expected to increase as quickly as the demand for services. Rather than hiring other dentists, current dental practitioners are more likely to hire dental assistants or dental hygienists to perform routine procedures.

According to the OOH, employment of dentists is expected to grow slower than the average for all occupations through 2006. Some employment growth is expected. The largest number of job openings will be created as a result of the expected retirement of a large number of dentists.

In spite of the rather guarded outlook for employment of dentists in general, practicing holistic dentists project that employment for holistic dentists will grow faster due to the increasing acceptance of the general public.

Holistic dentists expect growth in their field to be at least about as fast as the average. The national movement toward alternative health care therapies is likely to bring an even greater demand for holistic dentists.

For More Information

For comprehensive general information about the practice of dentistry in the United States, information on state an local dental organizations, and on the American Student Dental Association contact:

American Dental Association
211 East Chicago Avenue
Chicago, Illinois 60611
Tel: 312-440-2500
Web: http://www.ada.org

For an introduction to the field and philosophy of holistic dentistry and a searchable database of members, visit:

Holistic Dental Association
PO Box 5007
Durango, CO 81301
Email: hda@frontier.net
Web: http://www.holisticdental.org

For articles on holistic health, self-help resources in the United States, and a searchable database of practitioner members, contact:

American Holistic Health Association (AHHA)
PO Box 17400, Department R
Anaheim, CA 92817-7400
Tel: 714-779-6152
Email: ahha@healthy.net
Web: http://ahha.org

Holistic Physicians

School Subjects
Biology
Business
Chemistry

Personal Skills
Helping/teaching
Technical/scientific

Work Environment
Primarily indoors
Primarily multiple locations

Minimum Education Level
Medical degree

Salary Range
$32,789 to $160,000 to $238,000

Certification or Licensing
Required by all states

Outlook
Faster than the average

Overview

Holistic physicians are licensed medical doctors who embrace the philosophy of treating the patient as a whole person. Their goal is to help the individual achieve maximum well-being for the mind, body, and spirit. Holistic medicine emphasizes a cooperative relationship between physician and patient and focuses on educating patients in taking responsibility for their lives and their health. Holistic physicians use many approaches to diagnosis and treatment, including many other alternative approaches, such as acupuncture, meditation, nutritional counseling, and lifestyle changes. They also use drugs and surgery when no less invasive treatments can be found. Holistic physicians are part of the rapidly growing field of alternative health care practitioners. Most work in private practice or in alternative health clinics.

History

As much as 5,000 years ago, healing traditions of ancient cultures, such as China and India, promoted living a healthy life in harmony with nature. From 500 BC to AD 300, temples were major sources of physical and emotional healing in the Near East, the Mediterranean, and throughout Europe. It is reported that in these healing temples, the mind and body of the individual were treated together as a whole.

In the 4th century BC, Socrates postulated that the whole must be well in order for a part of the whole to be well. Hippocrates, who is sometimes considered to be the father of Western medicine, taught his students to assess the living environment of their patients in order to understand their illnesses.

The modern term "holism" was first used in 1926 by Jan Smuts in his book *Holism and Evolution*. Smuts championed the idea that living things are much more than just the sum of their parts. He challenged the views of modern medical science, which reduced the individual to a collection of body parts and diseases and denied the complexity of the human experience.

During the middle of the 20th century, scientific medical advances focused on germs—outside sources of disease. Now there was an enemy to fight, and the war on disease was fought with drugs to kill the microscopic invaders. Being healthy became a matter of overcoming disease, and people looked to modern medicine to cure their ills. For a time, holistic health concepts fell out of favor in the United States.

Dr. Evart Loomis is considered by many to be the "father of holistic medicine." As early as 1940, Dr. Loomis believed that all aspects of an individual had to be considered in order to determine the cause of an illness. In 1958, he and his wife, Vera, founded Meadowlark, thought to be the first holistic medical retreat center in the United States.

In the late 1950s and early 1960s, the holistic medical movement began to grow as people became increasingly aware that modern medicine did not have all the answers. Many chronic (long-term) conditions did not respond to medical treatment. Some side effects and cures even proved to be worse than the diseases. By the 1970s, "holistic" had become a common term. During the last decades of the 20th century, the use of holistic principles was increasingly incorporated into individual lifestyles and into the practice of medicine.

The Job

In many ways, the primary duties of holistic physicians are much like those of allopathic physicians (conventional doctors). They care for the sick and injured and counsel patients on preventive health care. They take medical histories, examine patients, and diagnose illnesses. Holistic physicians also prescribe and perform diagnostic tests and prescribe medications. They may refer patients to specialists and other health care providers as needed. They use conventional drugs and surgery when less invasive approaches are not appropriate or effective.

An important difference between the practices of allopathic physicians and holistic physicians is the approach to the patient/doctor relationship. Holistic doctors work in partnership with their patients. To establish a partnership relationship, holistic practitioners usually spend more time with their clients than allopathic doctors do. The initial visit for an allopathic practitioner is usually 20 to 30 minutes; holistic doctors usually spend 45 minutes to an hour or more on an initial visit. For conventional physicians, most follow-up visits average 7 to 10 minutes, while holistic practitioners take 30 to 45 minutes for the same visits.

During the initial history and physical, holistic physicians ask questions about all aspects of a person's life—not just the immediate symptoms of illness. If holistic practitioners are trained in homeopathy, the interview will be particularly detailed. They want to know about what you eat, how you sleep, what your life is like, what your stresses are, what makes you happy or sad, what your goals and beliefs are, and much more. They also ask about your family health history and your health. Holistic physicians don't just want to know today's symptoms. They try to find the underlying causes of those symptoms. They listen very carefully, and they do not make personal judgments about their patients' lives. They strive to have an attitude of unconditional positive regard for and acceptance of their patients.

Holistic physicians believe that maintaining health is the best approach to eliminating illness. They discuss your lifestyle with you, and discuss suggestions for ways you can work together to improve your health and your life. Nutrition and exercise are often important components of your wellness program.

Holistic doctors use healing modalities that consider the whole person and support the body's natural healing capabilities. They use a variety of approaches to diagnosis and treatment. For chronic (long-term) problems, they frequently recommend natural methods of treatment that have been shown to be more effective than conventional approaches. They are usually trained in several alternative health modalities themselves, but they may refer you to a specialist in another area if their expertise in that approach is not adequate for your needs. For example, a holistic practitioner may be trained in homeopathy, but not in acupuncture. If you would benefit from acupuncture for arthritis, the holistic physician will refer you for treatment.

Like other physicians, holistic practitioners utilize conventional drugs, laboratory tests, or surgery when necessary. They discuss the drugs, tests, or other procedures with you in advance. They answer your questions and help you understand your options. Holistic physicians give you choices and involve you in decisions about your healing program.

In addition to their regular duties as health care providers, holistic physicians must complete an enormous amount of paperwork. Whether they work in clinics or in private practice, they keep accurate patient records. More and more insurance companies are covering alternative services that are performed by licensed physicians. Holistic practitioners must frequently submit records to insurance companies in order to be paid for their services.

Those who work in private practice must also supervise the operations of their practices. This can involve interviewing, hiring, and training. Physicians in private practice may spend a large percentage of their time on business matters.

Requirements

High School

To become a holistic physician, you will have to study for 11 to 18 years after high school. Preparing for this profession is extremely demanding. Because you'll be entering a premed program in college, you'll want to take as many science classes as you can. Biology, chemistry, and physics will prepare you for college medical courses.

Holistic physicians need excellent communication abilities in order to build successful partnership relationships with their patients. Psychology, English, speech, and debate can help sharpen your communication skills. Business, mathematics, and computer courses can help you gain the skills you need to be a successful businessperson.

Postsecondary Training

To become a holistic physician, you must first become a conventional physician. That takes many years of study and training. First, you earn your bachelor's degree. Premedical students must take undergraduate courses in biology, organic and inorganic chemistry, physics, English, and mathematics.

There is strong competition for acceptance to medical school. Once you are accepted, you will spend four years in medical school. During the first two years, you will study anatomy, biochemistry, microbiology, psychology, medical ethics, pathology, pharmacology, and medical law. You will spend a lot of time in science laboratories. During the last two years, you will work in hospitals and clinics. Experienced physicians will supervise you as you work with patients and learn about medical specialties, such as family practice, internal medicine, pediatrics, and surgery. After completing medical school, you will have three to eight years of internship and residency, depending on your chosen specialty.

At the present time, training for competency in holistic or alternative medicine is not a part of regular medical training. At the insistence of many students, nearly a third of all conventional medical schools now include courses in alternative therapies, but they are still relatively few in number. As the interest in alternative approaches grows, the number of courses available in medical schools will undoubtedly increase. Most holistic physicians train themselves in alternative modalities through special postgraduate work and continuing education. A few graduate schools now offer specialized programs in alternative health care approaches and a very few residencies are available.

Certification or Licensing

All 50 states, the District of Columbia, and the U.S. territories license physicians. To obtain a license, you must graduate from an accredited medical school. You must also pass a licensing exam and complete one to seven years of graduate medical education.

At this time, there is no special certification or licensing available for holistic physicians. A practitioner's decision to use the term "holistic physician" or "alternative physician" is strictly voluntary. The American Holistic Medical Association (AHMA) established the American Board of Holistic Medicine (ABHM) in 1996. The ABHM has developed a core curriculum on which it will base board certification for holistic physicians. A certificate indicates that an individual has met the voluntary education and testing requirements of a particular certifying organization.

Other Requirements

To be a holistic physician, the whole-person approach to healing must be an integral part of your belief system and your life. You must have a fundamental respect for the dignity of humankind and a strong desire to help others.

Excellent listening, communication, and observational skills are essential. You also need the ability to make quick, good critical judgements and decisions in emergencies. Practicing holistic medicine requires an open mind and a commitment to lifelong learning.

Holistic physicians must be highly self-motivated and have the stamina to survive long hours and pressures of education and practice. You need to have the courage of your convictions and enjoy trail blazing. Even though alternative health care approaches have become more respected within the medical community in recent years, many physicians still do not accept them. Idealism and high ethical standards are essential. Most holistic physicians also need excellent business skills to run their own practices.

Exploring

Since the study of medicine involves such a long, expensive educational process, it is a good idea to explore the field carefully in advance to decide whether a career as a holistic physician is for you. Join science clubs and design projects relating to medicine and health care.

Visit your local health food stores and explore the nutrition and homeopathic sections. Talk with the staff. You may find some very knowledgeable, helpful people. Pick up any alternative newspapers and magazines they have. Volunteer at a hospital or nursing home to see how you feel about working with people who are sick or injured.

Contact the professional associations listed at the end of this article for information. Consider joining as a student member. The Internet has a wealth of information. Some Web sites have chat groups; others have searchable databases. You can ask questions and receive answers from some very prominent people in the field of alternative health care.

The Web sites of the professional associations have searchable databases of holistic physicians. Find one in your area and make an appointment for a physical exam. Experience how the practitioner works and consider whether you would like to practice medicine this way. Ask the physician about the field. Perhaps that person would be willing to hire you for a summer or part-time position or become your mentor.

Employers

The major employers of holistic physicians are physicians who have large practices, group practices, or alternative health clinics. An increasing number of physicians become partners or salaried employees of group practices. Working with a medical group spreads out the cost of medical equipment and other business expenses. In response to public interest and use of alternative approaches, a number of hospitals are opening alternative health care centers.

Some holistic physicians practice privately or with a partner. More holistic physicians are currently practicing on the East Coast and the West Coast in areas where alternative health care is already more accepted. The demand for holistic physicians is growing in all areas of the country.

Starting Out

The medical school you attend will have listings for job openings for physicians. If you have established a particular rapport with a staff member, that person might be able to help you. Professional journals, daily newspapers, and the Internet also have listings.

Networking is one of the best ways to find employment. Join professional organizations, attend meetings, and get to know people in the field. Networking with others in your field gives you a better chance of getting to know physicians who share some of your philosophies about holistic health.

Working in the practice or clinic of another physician who shares your beliefs about the practice of medicine is one of the best ways to get started as a holistic physician. It is hard to learn in isolation. When you interview potential employers, learn about their approaches to medicine. Be sure the setting will help you apply the skills you have learned without compromising what you believe about good health care.

A few holistic physicians go into private practice right away. Some set up a new practice, while others purchase an established practice from a physician who is retiring or moving.

Advancement

Holistic physicians can advance in a variety of ways. One who starts out as a salaried employee in a large practice or clinic may eventually become a partner. Holistic practitioners also advance by building their clientele and setting up their own practices or group practices. They sometimes buy the practices of retiring practitioners to add to their own.

Another avenue for advancement is specialization. Holistic practitioners may specialize in traditional medical specialties, such as pediatrics or obstetrics and gynecology, or they may choose to specialize in an area of alternative medicine, such as acupuncture or homeopathy.

For holistic physicians, continuing education is an important part of advancement. Holistic health care requires even more continual learning than conventional medicine. You will want to keep up on developments in the alternative modalities that interest you most, such as homeopathy, herbal therapy, Oriental medicine, or nutrition. And of course, you will have to keep current on changes in conventional medicine.

Teaching, writing, and public speaking are yet other directions for professional improvement. A few holistic physicians become executives with state or national organizations, such as the National Committee on Complementary and Alternative Medicine (NCCAM).

Earnings

Holistic physicians generally earn about as much as allopathic physicians who work in the same settings. According to the Association of American Medical Colleges, in 1996-1997 salaries of medical residents averaged from $32,789 to $40,849, depending on years of experience. According to the 1998-99 *Occupational Outlook Handbook*, the median net income of conventional physicians was around $160,000 per year in 1995. Physicians who worked in specialties had the highest earnings. Radiologists topped the list at $230,000. Of course, earnings vary according to experience, skill, hours worked, geographic region, and many other factors.

Some holistic practitioners may earn less because they spend more time with their patients, so they can see fewer in a day. Some make up the difference by charging more per visit. Others may earn less because they work fewer hours or days—in keeping with their belief in the importance of a balanced lifestyle. Holistic physicians tend to work between 40 and 50 hours a week, while their conventional counterparts work 50 to 60 hours or more.

Benefits vary according to the position of the physician. Those who work for large practices, clinics, or hospitals may receive benefit packages that include sick pay, vacation time, insurance, and other benefits. Those who are partners in a practice or are self-employed must provide their own benefits.

Work Environment

Holistic physicians work in particularly clean, quiet, comfortable surroundings. In keeping with their emphasis on whole-person relationships, many believe making their offices or clinics comfortable and pleasant is of particular importance. They may use air filtration systems and aromatherapy and choose ergonomically appropriate furniture and work stations.

Most group practices and solo practitioners have an office suite. The suite generally has a reception area. In clinics, several professionals may share this area. Most holistic physicians have a secretary or office staff. The suite also contains examining rooms and treatment rooms. In a clinic where several professionals work, there are usually separate offices for the individual professionals.

Holistic physicians who work in large practices or clinics need to work well in a group environment. They may work under supervision or in a team with other professionals. Those who work alone need a lot of self-discipline and must be highly motivated.

Most holistic physicians work four to five days a week. Some work 40 hours a week, although others put in longer hours. Larger practices and clinics may determine the hours of work, but holistic physicians in private practice can set their own. Evening and weekend hours may be scheduled to accommodate patients' needs. Physicians frequently travel between office and hospital to care for their patients.

Outlook

The 1998-99 *Occupational Outlook Handbook* (OOH) predicts that employment for physicians will grow faster than the average for all occupations through the year 2006. Demand for holistic physicians can be expected to keep pace with or exceed the demand for conventional physicians due to the recent rapid growth in interest in alternative health care approaches.

Rising health care costs have caused the country to reexamine the health care system. As efforts to control health care costs increase, the general public, the government, and the insurance industry will turn more and more to physicians who provide cost-effective, quality health care services.

Employment opportunities are expected to be best for primary care physicians, including general and family practitioners, general internists, and general pediatricians. Preventive care specialists and geriatric specialists will be in demand; these are areas in which holistic physicians excel.

According to the *Occupational Outlook Handbook,* highly respected sources indicate there is currently an oversupply of physicians. The OOH projects that the oversupply could result in physicians having to practice in underserved areas, working fewer hours, and having lower earnings. Opportunities in rural and lower-income areas should be good.

For More Information

For articles on holistic health, self-help resources in the United States, and a searchable database of practitioner members, contact:

American Holistic Health Association (AHHA)
PO Box 17400, Department R
Anaheim, CA 92817-7400
Tel: 714-779-6152
Web: http://ahha.org

For principals of holistic medical practice, the proposed board certification for holistic medicine, and a searchable database of members, contact:

American Holistic Medical Association (AHMA)
6728 Old McLean Village Drive
McLean, VA 22101
Tel: 703-556-9728
Web: http://www.holisticmedicine.org

Homeopaths

School Subjects
Biology
Chemistry
English

Personal Skills
Helping/teaching
Technical/scientific

Work Environment
Primarily indoors
Primarily one location

Minimum Education Level
Some postsecondary training

Salary Range
$30,000 to $90,000 to $175,000

Certification or Licensing
Required by certain states

Outlook
Much faster than the average

Overview

Samuel Hahnemann, the founder of homeopathy, said, "The highest ideal of cure is the speedy, gentle, and enduring restoration of health by the most trustworthy and least harmful way." *Homeopaths* are health care professionals who practice a complete system of natural medicine called *homeopathy*. Homeopathic care generally costs less than conventional medical care, and homeopathic medicine is safe, effective, and natural. Homeopathy is used to maintain good health and to treat acute as well as chronic ailments. It has proven to be effective in many instances where conventional medicines have been unsuccessful. Some of its remedies are simple enough to be used by people who are not medically trained.

Homeopathy is part of the rapidly growing field of alternative/complementary health care. Unlike conventional medicine, it does not treat just the symptoms of a disease. Instead, it seeks the underlying cause of the illness. It seeks to stimulate the patient's natural defenses and the immune system so the body can heal itself. Homeopaths believe that being healthy means being balanced mentally, emotionally, and physically. In this sense, homeopathy is truly a holistic medical model. The presently popular concept of health maintenance is not new to homeopathy. It is what homeopaths have been practicing for nearly 200 years. In 1998, more than 3,000 homeopaths were working in the United States. Most homeopathic practitioners work in private practice, but some work in clinics with other health care professionals.

History

The history of homeopathy is one of struggle and excitement. Samuel Hahnemann, a renowned German physician, founded homeopathy nearly 200 years ago. Medical practices in the 1700s and 1800s often caused more harm than good. Physicians routinely used bloodletting, purging, and large doses of toxic medicines as part of their treatments. Dr. Hahnemann wanted to find a more humane approach. Through years of careful observation, experimentation, and documentation, he developed the system of medicine that he named homeopathy. Homeopathy grew because it was systematic, effective, and comparatively inexpensive. Precisely because of its benefits, the new system threatened the medical establishment. Dr. Hahnemann was persecuted and even arrested. However, he was determined and courageous, and he continued his work throughout his life. His system of medicine spread throughout the world.

Several doctors who had studied homeopathy in Europe emigrated to the United States around 1825. They introduced homeopathy to other physicians, and its popularity grew rapidly. By the mid-1800s, several medical colleges in the United States taught homeopathy. In 1844, homeopaths established the first national medical society in America—the American Institute of Homeopathy. The practice of homeopathy continued to thrive until the early 1900s. At the turn of the century, the United States had 22 homeopathic medical colleges, and one-fifth of the country's medical doctors used homeopathy.

However, like Samuel Hahnemann in Europe, the homeopaths in the United States seemed to pose a threat to the conventional medical and pharmaceutical establishments. For a variety of reasons—attacks by the medical establishment, growth in popularity of a more "mechanical" model of medicine, and discord among homeopaths themselves—the practice of homeopathy in the United States declined. By the late 1940s, there were no homeopathy courses in this country.

Homeopaths in other countries also experienced opposition. However, homeopathy flourished wherever people were allowed to practice it with relative freedom. Today, over 500 million people worldwide receive homeopathic treatment. Homeopathy is popular in England, France, Germany, the Netherlands, India, Pakistan, Sri Lanka, Brazil, and many other countries.

Because homeopathic treatments and drugs are natural and relatively inexpensive, even countries with limited resources can take advantage of them. In this country, there has been a tremendous increase in interest in homeopathy since the 1970s. Statistics show that Americans are turning to this form of treatment in dramatic numbers. As alternative health care is growing, so is the field of homeopathy.

The Job

Homeopaths help people improve their lives and get well. They look at illness differently than conventional doctors do. They view the symptoms of an illness as the body's attempts to heal itself. For example, they see a cough as the body's efforts to rid itself of something that is foreign to the system. Instead of trying to suppress the symptoms, homeopaths search for the underlying cause of the problem. They try to discover the more fundamental reason for the illness. Why was the body susceptible to a cough in the first place?

To homeopaths, people are healthy when their lives are balanced mentally, emotionally, and physically. If any aspect of the patient's life is out of balance, it could lead to illness. A symptom, such as a cough, is just the top layer of a problem, and homeopaths work to peel away all the layers and get to the root of the problem. The goal of homeopathic medicine is not just to cure the ailment, but rather to return the individual to optimum health.

To discover the reasons for an illness, homeopaths begin with a very detailed individual interview. The first interview usually takes at least an hour and may last up to two hours. Homeopathic treatment is based entirely on the individual. Homeopaths believe that every person is unique and that individuals experience the same illness differently. Although two people may complain of a "cold," each of them will have unique symptoms and be affected in different ways. The homeopathic practitioner asks questions about every aspect of the individual's life—health symptoms, eating habits, sleeping patterns, reactions to heat and chill, and so on. In order to process all of this information, homeopaths must have good communication and analytical skills and be very attentive to detail. Choosing the right cure depends on understanding every aspect of the individual's situation, not just the illness.

To help guide their research, homeopaths classify people into categories called *constitutional types*. They determine an individual's constitutional type according temperament, physical appearance, emotional history, previous ailments, preferences about food, reactions to the weather, and many other traits. Then they search for a constitutional medicine—one that produces symptoms that are most similar to the individual's symptoms.

Homeopathy is based upon the principle that "like cures like" (the Law of Similars). Dr. Hahnemann observed that a substance that produces the symptoms of an illness when given in a large dose could cure the illness if it were given in a minute dose. The theory is that the small dose stimulates the body's natural healing power to fight off the illness. Hippocrates, the Greek physician who is considered to be the father of medicine, first recognized this principle in 4 BC. The Law of Similars is also the theory behind some conventional medicines, such as the vaccine that prevents polio and the treatment of allergies.

After determining the individual's constitutional type, homeopaths seek out the substance that is capable of producing the same symptoms that the individual is experiencing. They can spend much of their day at the office studying their notes and researching. They search through books called *repertories* or use computers to find the right constitutional medicine.

Homeopaths use very small doses of natural medicines to stimulate the body to heal itself. The Law of the Infinitesimal Dose is another important principle of homeopathic medicine. It states that the more dilute a remedy is, the more powerful it is. Although this seems paradoxical, years of clinical study have shown the small doses to be effective.

Homeopathic medicines are natural, safe, and effective. They are specially prepared from plant, animal, or mineral extracts. The raw material is dissolved in a mixture of alcohol and water. Then it is diluted several times and shaken vigorously. The Food and Drug Administration (FDA) recognizes homeopathic remedies as official drugs. It regulates their production, labeling, and distribution just as it does conventional medicines. Homeopathic remedies are collected in an official compendium, the *Homeopathic Pharmacopoeia of the United States*, which was first published in 1894.

After homeopaths choose a remedy, they instruct the individual in its use. This may happen at the end of the initial interview if the person's symptoms point to an obvious cure. Many times however, homeopaths must spend a long time searching for the remedy that matches the essence of the person's symptoms. When that is the case, they may not give the individual a remedy at the first session. Finding the exact constitutional medicine requires patience, experience, problem-solving ability, and intuition.

The course of treatment depends on the individual's circumstances, symptoms, and prognosis. After a prescribed period of time, the individual generally returns for a follow-up visit. This visit typically lasts from 15 to 45 minutes. During this time, homeopaths look for signs of improvement and sometimes choose a different remedy if the desired result has not been obtained. Usually only one remedy is given at a time because the goal is to stimulate the body's natural defenses with a minimal amount of medicine.

Homeopaths tend to discourage frequent visits unless they are medically necessary. The time between visits is usually from one to six months.

Most homeopaths work in private practice, so they must know how to handle all of the paperwork and run the business. Many are health care professionals who are licensed in other medical fields, such as acupuncturists, chiropractors, physicians, naturopaths, nurse practitioners, and osteopaths. Licensed professionals must understand and manage their own malpractice insurance and their patients' insurance claims. More and more insurance policies cover visits to homeopaths who are also licensed health practitioners. If homeopaths are not licensed, insurance will probably not cover their treatments. The use of the computer is becoming increasingly important to homeopaths. The collected wisdom of centuries of homeopathy is rapidly being made available in computerized databases, and this is an invaluable aid to the arduous research of the homeopath.

Homeopathic practitioners are usually highly dedicated individuals. As Sharon Stevenson, Executive Director of the National Center for Homeopathy put it, "Once they catch the 'fever' they just can't help themselves. They get satisfaction from working with a kind of medicine that really cures and doesn't just cover up illness. And the medicines aren't going to make the patients sick." Homeopaths believe strongly in the benefits homeopathic care can bring to their patients and to the world. They have the great reward of helping people and seeing them get well. In addition to their practices, many homeopaths are involved in the effort to expand the understanding and acceptance of homeopathy throughout the country. They participate in research and give lectures. Some are involved in politics fighting for legislation to benefit homeopathy.

Requirements

High School

People from many different backgrounds practice homeopathy. Most homeopaths in the United States are licensed health professionals. Among them, medical doctors are the majority. Many other licensed professionals, such as acupuncturists, chiropractors, naturopaths, medical assistants, nurse practitioners, and nurses also specialize in homeopathy. In addition, there is a small group of practitioners of homeopathy who do not have licenses in a health care field. The basic skills, interests, and talents required to be a good homeopath are common to all of these professionals, but educational requirements differ according to the individual health field.

Because of its medical nature, homeopathy requires a solid background in the sciences. Biology and chemistry will help you prepare for a career in homeopathy. The emphasis on careful interviews and detailed documentation make English, journalism, speech, debate, psychology, and sociology classes very valuable. Since most homeopaths are solo practitioners, business and computer courses are also recommended. The basics learned in high school will allow you to become familiar with standard medical knowledge and to use this information as a foundation for in-depth study of homeopathy.

Postsecondary Training

If a career in homeopathy interests you, there are many paths from which to choose. Most future homeopaths study health-related fields in college, for example, nutrition, biology, premed, or nursing. Careers such as nutritionist, medical assistant, and nurse require fewer years of training to become licensed. Others, like chiropractor, naturopathic physician, or physician require considerably more years of study. The specific courses you need will depend upon your choice of health field. Some particularly beneficial areas of study include: anatomy, physiology, and disease and pathology. In many cases, individuals complete their studies for their licenses and then take courses in homeopathy that are offered at several institutions around the country.

After college, some future homeopaths go to medical school. There is a growing interest in homeopathy among physicians, and homeopaths are working toward integrating homeopathy into the curricula of conventional medical schools.

Another path toward a career in homeopathy is to earn a doctorate in naturopathic medicine. Naturopathic medicine is an approach to natural healing that incorporates an array of healing modalities, including homeopathy. There are four naturopathic medical schools in North America. They offer four-year programs with homeopathy as a specialty. These schools require at least two years of chemistry, a year of biology, and some other premedical coursework prior to admission.

It is easier to practice homeopathy if you are also licensed to practice conventional or naturopathic medicine. However, there are some programs for those who are not medically trained. Training in homeopathy can demand as much time and effort as medical studies. Programs are available on a part-time basis for those who need flexible class hours. There are also a few respected correspondence courses. If you are interested in studying abroad, England, India, and France have schools for classical homeopathy.

There are no federally funded programs for student aid for homeopathy. Some of the professional societies do offer scholarships or other assistance. If you are seriously considering a career in homeopathy, contact the national homeopathic associations listed at the end of this article for information about programs, requirements, and scholarship funds.

Certification or Licensing

Certification indicates that a homeopath has met the standards of education and knowledge set by a particular professional association. An individual can be a certified homeopath but still not be licensed to practice medicine. Licensing is a requirement established by government. Homeopaths who are licensed health care practitioners in other fields, such as chiropractors, physicians, naturopathic physicians, nurses, and nurse practitioners, must maintain the appropriate licenses for their specific fields.

Both certification and licensing requirements for homeopaths vary according to state. Some states do not consider homeopathy to be the practice of medicine, so they do not regulate its practice. Other states require homeopaths to be licensed in some other form of health care. Arizona, Connecticut, and Nevada offer homeopathic medical licenses. Check with the office of the attorney general in your state to be sure you know its certification and licensing requirements. Although some homeopaths currently practice without a medical license, professionals in the field agree that the trend is toward certification and licensing. If you are interested in a career in homeopathy, it is recommended that you acquire a license in some related field of medicine.

Other Requirements

To be a successful homeopath, you need to enjoy helping and working with people. On the other hand, you must also be self-motivated and enjoy researching and working alone. You need to be inquisitive, detail oriented, independent, and self-reliant. It helps to enjoy solving mysteries and puzzles.

In addition, you must know your own mind and have the courage of your convictions. Because homeopathy is re-emerging as an important form of alternative health care in this country, homeopaths need to have strong convictions and be able to take criticism. They may have to defend their work or try to educate others who know little about homeopathy. It helps for a homeopath to be a bit of a crusader.

Exploring

There are many ways for you to learn about homeopathy right now. Ask your librarian for homeopathic journals, newsletters, and books. Visit your local health food stores and explore the homeopathic section. Talk with the staff. You may find some very knowledgeable, helpful people. Pick up any alternative newspapers and magazines they have. Ask if there are homeopathic practitioners or pharmacists in the area. If there are, visit them, and talk to them about their work. There are still relatively few homeopaths in this country, but they are generally enthusiastic supporters of others who are interested in the career. Check the Internet. There is a wealth of information online, and there are alternative medicine/holistic health forums where you can discuss homeopathic medicine with people in the field. If possible, make an appointment with a homeopath so you can experience this approach to health care for yourself.

The National Center for Homeopathy has 160 affiliated study groups throughout the country where beginners can study. These are groups of lay people who meet once or twice a month to study homeopathy together. The National Center for Homeopathy also offers summer programs where you can study a variety of topics and live and learn with others interested in the field—from beginners to experts. Sharon Stevenson says of the summer programs, "They are a wonderful, intensive experience where you get to rub elbows with homeopaths from all over the country. You live in a dorm, study, eat, and relax together. Bonds are formed that last a lifetime."

Employers

Most homeopaths practice on their own or with a partner. Working with a partner makes practicing easier because the costs of running an office are shared. Other tasks, such as bookkeeping and record keeping can also be shared. Alternative health clinics and some other health care professionals may hire homeopaths. Hospitals and other health care agencies generally do not hire homeopaths, but they may as the alternative health care movement grows.

It is easier to practice homeopathy in some areas of the United States, such as on the West Coast and in larger cities, but there are practicing homeopaths throughout the country.

Starting Out

Since homeopaths come from so many different backgrounds, ways to get started vary, too. Licensed professionals generally begin practicing the discipline in which they are licensed. Some build their homeopathic practice along with the other practice. Others just begin a homeopathic practice. Unlicensed homeopaths may work with licensed individuals. In these cases, the licensed professional is generally legally responsible for the work of the unlicensed homeopath. Some unlicensed individuals have been known to offer their services for free at the beginning, just to gain experience.

Homeopathy is a growing field, but it is still a relatively small community of professionals. Once you get to know others in the field, you may be able to find a mentor who will help you learn how to get started. Networking with others in the field can be an extremely valuable way to learn and grow.

Advancement

Advancement comes with building a solid reputation. Homeopaths whose practices grow may eventually need to look for partners in order to take care of more patients. Many homeopaths are active promoters of the discipline. They write articles for journals or magazines or present information on homeopathy in public forums, such as on radio and television.

Others pursue research into homeopathic treatments and present their findings to colleagues at conventions or publish their work in the homeopathic journals. A few may work with the homeopathic pharmaceutical companies.

Earnings

Since so many homeopaths are in solo practice, incomes vary widely according to the number of hours worked and the rates charged. Statistics on earnings in the field are not yet available, but homeopathic professionals tend to agree that homeopathic physicians charge between $100 and $300 for an initial visit of 60 to 90 minutes and $50 to$100 for a follow-up visit of 15 to 45 minutes. Unlicensed homeopaths charge between $50 and $250 for the same initial visit and $30 to $80 for a follow-up. They may take several years to build a practice, and their rates will usually remain on the lower end of the scale. Fees tend to increase the longer the individual has been practicing.

According to Dana Ullman, nationally known author of several books on homeopathy, licensed professionals earn about the average for their professions or a little less. For example, homeopathic physicians earn $90,000 to $175,000 a year. They have good incomes, but generally not as high as the average medical doctor. Other licensed professionals, such as homeopathic nurses, might earn $60,000 to $100,000. Unlicensed homeopaths usually earn less, perhaps beginning around $30,000. As with all self-employed individuals, income is directly related to number of hours worked and fees charged.

Since most homeopaths are solo practitioners, they must supply their own benefits, such as vacations, insurance, and retirement funds. In addition, licensed professionals must maintain their licenses and pay for their own malpractice insurance.

Work Environment

Homeopaths work indoors, usually in their own offices, and sometimes even in their homes. As a result, they have the surroundings of their choice. Since they meet with patients and also spend time in research, they frequently have quiet, pleasant offices. Most work on their own with little, if any, supervision, so it is important for them to be self-motivated. Many homeopaths also have the ability to determine the number of hours and days they work per week. They may set schedules that make it easy for their patients to make appointments.

Outlook

The field of homeopathy is growing rapidly along with the national interest in alternative health care. According to a 1997 survey of American Medical Association members, nearly 50 percent of the doctors who participated in the survey indicated an interest in homeopathic training. In a 1998 interview, Ms. Stevenson of the National Center for Homeopathy stated that there was a shortage of trained homeopaths, and many established homeopathic practitioners had waiting lists ranging from two months to one years.

Homeopathy can be combined with a variety of health care professions. Many practitioners include it among other healing approaches they use. However, many homeopaths believe that it is best to specialize in homeopathy. The amount of experience and the complexity of the knowledge required to become a good practitioner make homeopathy a lifelong education.

The World Health Organization (WHO), the medical branch of the United Nations, cited homeopathy as one of the systems of traditional medicine that should be integrated worldwide with conventional medicine in order to provide adequate global health care in the next century. The field of homeopathy is growing much faster than the average. According to Dana Ullman, "Homeopathy is not mainstream medicine. It is on the cutting edge of medicine and healing. If you are good at homeopathy, you will always have plenty of patients, and you will be in demand anywhere in the world."

For More Information

This national organization certifies practitioners of classical homeopathy:

Council for Homeopathic Certification
1199 Sanchez Street
San Francisco, CA 94114
Tel: 415-789-7677
Web: http://www.healthy.net/othersites/homeopathiccouncil

This professional association provides education and training for homeopathic professionals and for interested consumers who want to learn homeopathy for their own use.

National Center for Homeopathy
801 North Fairfax Street, Suite 306
Alexandria, VA 22314
Tel: 703-548-7790
Email: info@homeopathic.org
Web: http://homeopathic.org

For comprehensive Internet information on homeopathy as well as extensive links, visit:

Homeopathic Educational Services
http//www.homeopathic.com

Homeopathy Home
http//www.homeopathyhome.com

Kinesiologists

Health Physical education	School Subjects
Communication/ideas Helping/teaching	Personal Skills
Primarily indoors Primarily one location	Work Environment
Bachelor's degree	Minimum Education Level
$16,000 to $28,000 to $48,000	Salary Range
Recommended	Certification or Licensing
About as fast as the average	Outlook

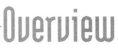

Overview

Kinesiologists (also known as *kinesiotherapists*) are health care workers who plan and conduct exercise programs to help their patients develop or maintain endurance, strength, mobility, and coordination. Many of their clients are people who have disabilities. They also work with patients who are recovering from injuries or illnesses and need help to keep their muscle tone during long periods of inactivity.

Kinesiology is based on the belief that each muscle in the body relates to a specific meridian—or energy pathway—in the body. These meridians also relate to organs, allowing the muscles to give us information about organ function and energy. The profession builds on basic principles from Chinese medicine, acupressure, and massage therapy to bring the body into balance. The goal is to release physical and mental pain, and alleviate tension in the mind and body. Relieving stress—be it physical, mental, emotional, chemical, environmental, or behavioral—is a main element of kinesiology. Various techniques are combined with visualization, massage, and movement exercises to help patients heal.

History

Kinesiology studies how the principles of mechanics and anatomy affect human movement. The word *kinesio* is derived from the Greek work *kinesis*, meaning motion. Kinesiology literally means the study of motion, or motion therapy. Kinesiology is based on the idea that physical education is a science.

Scientists throughout the centuries have studied how the body works: how muscles are connected, how bones grow, how blood flows. Kinesiology builds on all that knowledge. The practice of kinesiology developed during World War II, when physicians in military hospitals saw that appropriate exercise could help wounded patients heal faster and with better results than they'd had before. This exercise therapy proved particularly useful for injuries to the arms and legs.

By 1946, Veterans Administration hospitals were using prescribed exercise programs in rehabilitation treatment. Before long, other hospitals and clinics recognized the benefits of kinesiology and instituted similar programs. Within a few years the new therapy was an important part of many treatment programs, including programs for chronically disabled patients.

In the 1950s, a number of studies indicated that European children were more physically fit than American children were. To decrease the gap in fitness levels, the United States government instituted physical fitness programs in schools. This practical application of kinesiology to otherwise healthy children boosted the field dramatically.

Today, the study of physical fitness and the movement of the body is illustrated in countless fields. Although kinesiologists have historically worked with injured or disabled patients, as humans move towards a more computerized, less active lifestyle, kinesiologists and other health care professionals will be in higher demand to help people of all abilities maintain good health and fitness.

The Job

Kinesiology studies how muscles act and coordinate to move the body. Kinesiologists use muscle testing and physical therapy to evaluate and correct the state of various bodily functions in their patients. Kinesiologists take all body systems into account when treating a patient. And that is the most important aspect of kinesiology: its aim is to treat the patient, not to correct a disorder. Kinesiologists allow patients to work through a disability or disorder.

Kinesiologists work with a wide range of people, both individually and in groups. Their patients may be disabled children or adults, geriatric patients, psychiatric patients, the developmentally disabled, or amputees. Some may have had heart attacks, strokes, or spinal injuries. Others may be affected by such conditions as arthritis, impaired circulation, or cerebral palsy. Kinesiologists also work with people who were involved in automobile accidents, have congenital birth defects, or have sustained sports injuries.

These professionals work to help their clients be more self-reliant, enjoy leisure activities, and even adapt to new ways of living, working, and thriving. Although kinesiologists work with their patients physically, giving them constant encouragement and emotional support is also an important part of their work.

Kinesiologists' responsibilities may include teaching patients to use artificial limbs or walk with canes, crutches, or braces. They may help visually impaired people learn how to move around without help or teach patients who cannot walk how to drive cars with hand controls. For mentally ill people, therapists may develop therapeutic activities that help them release tension or teach them how to cooperate with others.

The work is often physically demanding. Kinesiologists work with such equipment as weights, pulleys, bikes, and rowing machines. They demonstrate exercises so their patients can learn to do them and also may teach members of their patients' families to help the patients exercise. They may work with their patients in swimming pools, whirlpools, saunas, or other therapeutic settings. When patients are very weak or have limited mobility, therapists may help them exercise by lifting them or moving their limbs.

Kinesiologists work as members of medical teams. Physicians describe the kind of exercise their patients should have, and then the therapists develop programs to meet the specific needs of the patients. Other members of the medical team may include nurses, psychologists, psychiatrists, social workers, massage therapists, physical therapists, acupuncturists, and vocational counselors.

Kinesiologists write reports on the clients' progress to provide necessary information for other members of the medical team. These reports, which describe the treatments and their results, may also provide useful information for researchers and other members of the health care team.

These therapists do not do the same work as physical therapists, orthotists, or prosthetists. *Physical therapists* test and measure the functions of the musculoskeletal, neurological, pulmonary, and cardiovascular systems and treat the problems that occur in these systems. *Orthotists* are concerned with supporting and bracing weak or ineffective joints and muscles, and *prosthetists* are concerned with replacing missing body parts with artificial devices. Kinesiologists focus instead on the interconnection of all these systems. In certain cases, they may refer a patient to another specialist for additional treatment.

Requirements

High School

High school students interested in this field should prepare for their college studies by taking a strong college-preparatory course load. Classes in anatomy, chemistry, biology, mathematics, and physics will give you the basic science background you will need to study kinesiology in college. Health, psychology, and social science will also be very helpful. Be sure to take physical education classes in order to gain a better appreciation for the nature of movement and our muscles. Participating in a sport will also help you learn more about kinesiology from an inside perspective.

Postsecondary Training

In order to practice kinesiology, you will need to earn a bachelor's degree from a four-year program at an accredited school. Some kinesiologists major in physical education and have kinesiology as a specialty, but a growing number of institutions in the United States are starting to offer undergraduate degrees in kinesiology. Kinesiology programs include classes in education, clinical practice, biological sciences, and behavioral sciences. Specific courses may have titles such as Movement Coordination, Control, and Skill; Performance and Physical Activity; Biomechanics; Motor Behavior; Exercise Physiology; and Exercise and Health Psychology. Master's degrees in kinesiology and related programs are currently offered at over 100 institutions; doctorates in the field can be earned at 55 universities.

After graduation, you will need to go on to a clinical internship, which generally consists of 1,000 hours of training at an approved health facility under the supervision of certified kinesiologists. You may also seek out an assistantship with a practicing kinesiologist.

Certification or Licensing

Although certification is not mandatory for every job, it is highly recommended as certification requirements are starting to become more regulated. Certification in kinesiology or kinesiotherapy requires a bachelor's degree in the specified accredited courses, 1,000 hours of clinical practice, and successful completion of an examination administered by the Commission on Accreditation of Allied Health Education Programs (CAAHEP). To take the examination, applicants must also be members of the American Kinesiotherapy Association.

After meeting the basic requirements and passing the examination, candidates become nationally certified kinesiologists. If they have earned undergraduate degrees in physical education, they also may become state-certified physical education teachers after meeting the certification requirements for the state in which they plan to work.

Other Requirements

Kinesiologists must have maturity and objectivity and should be able to work well with patients and other staff members. They must have excellent communication skills to explain the exercises so patients can understand their instructions and perform the exercises properly.

Kinesiologists need stamina to demonstrate the exercises and help patients with them. They need much patience since many exercise programs are repetitive and are carried out over long periods. A good sense of humor also helps to keep up patient morale. These professionals also must know how to plan and carry out their programs, and they must stay current on new developments in their field. Certification usually requires continuing education courses.

Exploring

If you are a high school student interested in this type of work, you can get experience in several ways. Basic physical education courses as well as team sports, like volleyball or track, will help you gain an appreciation for the possibilities and limitations of the body. Plan and carry out exercise programs, or instruct others in proper exercise techniques. Many exercise classes are often offered in scouting and by organizations such as the YMCA and YWCA.

Opportunities for volunteer, part-time, or summer work may be available at facilities that have kinesiology or kinesiotherapy programs, such as hospitals, clinics, nursing homes, and summer camps for disabled children. Health and exercise clubs also may have summer work or part-time jobs. In addition, you may be able to visit kinesiology departments at health care centers to talk with staff members and see how they work.

Employers

Kinesiologists work in many types of organizations. They work for the government in the Department of Veterans Affairs, public and private hospitals, sports medicine facilities, and rehabilitation facilities. Learning disability centers, grammar schools and high schools, colleges and universities, and health clubs also employ kinesiologists. Other kinesiologists work in private practice or as exercise consultants. Kinesiologists can also find employment with sports teams, or they may write for or edit sports, rehabilitative, and other medical journals. Many kinesiologists also teach in the field or do research.

Starting Out

The American Kinesiotherapy Association maintains an employment service for certified kinesiologists and kinesiotherapists. Plus, most colleges and universities offer job placement assistance for their alumni. Therapists also may apply at health facilities that have kinesiotherapy programs, including private and state hospitals, Department of Veterans Affairs hospitals, clinics, health clubs, chiropractic clinics, and rehabilitation centers. Many kinesiologists find employment by networking with other professionals in the field. Most professional organizations and associations maintain listings of positions open in various locations.

Beginning kinesiologists may gain paid employment with a facility if they start out doing volunteer work. Some organizations prefer to hire therapists with some work experience, and volunteer work gives the new kinesiotherapist a great opportunity to learn more about the field and a particular organization.

Advancement

Kinesiologists usually start as staff therapists at hospitals, clinics, or other health care facilities. After several years, they may become supervisors or department heads. Some move on to do consultant work for health care facilities. Some kinesiologists use their practical experience to do more research in the field, or they may teach at a kinesiology program. They may write for field newsletters or journals, reporting on their progress in rehabilitating a particular patient or in treating a specific disability. With advanced training, experienced kinesiologists may go on to more senior positions at health care centers, clinics, colleges, and related facilities.

Earnings

According to the American Kinesiotherapy Association, the average projected starting salary for registered kinesiotherapists is $28,000 per year. This, of course, depends on the experience of the kinesiologist and the location of the job. Since kinesiology is a relatively new field, few reliable salary sources exist, but salaries are probably comparable to related health professions.

According to the 1998-99 *Occupational Outlook Handbook*, occupational therapy assistants new to the field earned about $27,442 in 1995. Starting salaries for physical therapist assistants averaged about $24,000 per year in 1996. Those working in hospitals tended to earn less than those in private practice, who earned an average of about $30,000 in 1996. Average earnings of health aides, including physical therapist aides, were $16,000, while physical therapists earned approximately $48,000. Kinesiologist salaries are likely to be somewhere in those ranges.

Depending on their employers, most kinesiologists enjoy a full complement of benefits, including vacation and sick time as well as holidays and medical and dental insurance. Kinesiologists who work in a health care facility usually get free use of the equipment.

Work Environment

Kinesiologists who work in hospitals and clinics usually work a typical 40-hour workweek, with hours somewhere between 8:00 AM and 6:00 PM, Monday through Friday. Some may work evenings and weekends instead in order to accommodate their clients' schedules. Because of the long-range, rehabilitative nature of the work, most kinesiologists work a set schedule and generally don't have to be available for emergency situations.

The number of patients the therapist works with usually depends on the size and function of the facility. When leading a rehabilitation group, the kinesiologist may work with three to five patients at a time, helping them work on their own and as part of a team. Therapists may see their patients in hospitals and other health centers, or they may visit patients in their own homes, or arrange for rehabilitative outings. Their clients may be confined to beds, chairs, or wheelchairs. Exercises are often performed in pools or on ramps, stairways, or exercise tables.

Outlook

The employment outlook for kinesiologists and kinesiotherapists is expected to grow about as fast as the average for the next few years. The demand for their services may grow somewhat because of the increasing emphasis on services for disabled people, patients with specific disorders, and the growing number of older adults. Some medical workers also handle patients with chronic pain by using the physical rehabilitation and retraining at the base of kinesiology. Plus, kinesiology is certain to grow as a profession as more is learned about the field.

As health costs rise, the importance of outpatient care is expected to increase as well. Many insurance companies prefer to pay for home health care or outpatient care instead of lengthy, expensive—and often unnecessary—hospital stays. Part-time workers in the field will also see increased opportunities. In addition, openings will occur as many of the early kinesiotherapists reach retirement age and others change jobs or leave for other reasons.

For More Information

For more information about certification requirements, contact:

American Kinesiotherapy Association
Web: http://www.akta.org/

International College of Applied Kinesiology
6405 Metcalf Avenue, Suite 503
Shawnee Mission, KS 66202-3929
Tel: 913-384-5336
Web: http://www.icak.com/

The AAHPERD is an umbrella organization for a number of groups dedicated to health and fitness. For more detailed information on kinesiology and related fields, contact:

American Alliance for Health, Physical Education, Recreation and Dance
1900 Association Drive
Reston, VA 20191
Tel: 703-476-3400 or 1-800-213-7193
Web: http://www.aahperd.org/

American Physical Therapy Association
1111 North Fairfax Street
Alexandria, VA 22314
Tel: 703-684-2782
Web: http://www.apta.org/

Massage Therapists

Health Physical education	School Subjects
Helping/teaching Mechanical/manipulative	Personal Skills
Primarily indoors Primarily one location	Work Environment
Some postsecondary training	Minimum Education Level
$10,700 to $40,000 to $72,800	Salary Range
Required by certain states	Certification or Licensing
Faster than the average	Outlook

Overview

Massage therapy is a broad term referring to a number of health-related practices, including Swedish massage, sports massage, Rolfing, Shiatsu and acupressure, trigger point therapy, and reflexology. Although the techniques vary, most *massage therapists* (or *massotherapists*) press and rub the skin and muscles. Relaxed muscles, improved blood circulation and joint mobility, reduced stress and anxiety, and decreased recovery time for sprains and injured muscles are just a few of the potential benefits of massage therapy. Massage therapists are sometimes called *bodyworkers*. The titles *masseur* and *masseuse*, once common, are now rare among those who use massage for therapy and rehabilitation.

History

Getting a massage used to be considered a luxury reserved only for the very wealthy, or an occasional splurge for the less affluent. Some people thought massage to be a cover for illicit activities such as prostitution. With increased regulation of certification and a trend toward ergonomics in the home and workplace, however, massage therapy is recognized as an important tool in both alternative and preventative health care. Regular massage can help alleviate physical ailments faced by people today: physical stress brought on by an increase in sedentary lifestyle, aches and pains from hours spent in front of the computer, as well as injuries of the weekend warrior trying to make up for five days of inactivity.

The Job

Massage therapists work to produce physical, mental, and emotional benefits through the manipulation of the body's soft tissue. Auxiliary methods, such as the movement of joints and the application of dry and steam heat, are also used. Among the potential physical benefits are the release of muscle tension and stiffness, reduced blood pressure, better blood circulation, a shorter healing time for sprains and pulled muscles, increased flexibility and greater range of motion in the joints, and reduced swelling from edema (excess fluid buildup in body tissue). Massage may also improve posture, strengthen the immune system, and reduce the formation of scar tissue.

Mental and emotional benefits include a relaxed state of mind, reduced stress and anxiety, clearer thinking, and a general sense of well-being. Physical, mental, and emotional health are all interconnected: being physically fit and healthy can improve emotional health, just as a positive mental attitude can bolster the immune system to help the body fight off infection. A release of muscle tension also leads to reduced stress and anxiety, and physical manipulation of sore muscles can help speed the healing process.

There are many different approaches a massage therapist may take. Among the most popular are Swedish massage, sports massage, Rolfing, Shiatsu and acupressure, and trigger point therapy.

In Swedish massage the traditional techniques are effleurage, petrissage, friction, and tapotement. Effleurage (stroking), the use of light and hard rhythmic stroking movements, is used to relax muscles and improve blood circulation. It is often performed at the beginning and end of a massage session. Petrissage (kneading) is the rhythmic squeezing, pressing, and lifting of a muscle. For friction, the fingers, thumb, or palm or heel of the hand are pressed into the skin with a small circular movement. The massage therapist's fingers are sometimes pressed deeply into a joint. Tapotement (tapping), in which the hands strike the skin in rapid succession, is used to improve blood circulation. During the session the client, covered with sheets, lies undressed on a padded table. Oil or lotion is used to smooth the skin. Some massage therapists use aromatherapy, adding fragrant essences to the oil to relax the client and stimulate circulation. Swedish massage may employ a number of auxiliary techniques, including the use of rollers, belts, and vibrators; steam and dry heat; ultraviolet and infrared light; and saunas, whirlpools, steam baths, and packs of hot water or ice.

Sports massage is essentially Swedish massage used in the context of athletics. A light massage generally is given before an event or game to loosen and warm the muscles. This reduces the chance of injury and may improve performance. After the event the athlete is massaged more deeply to alleviate pain, reduce stiffness, and promote healing.

Rolfing, developed by American Ida Rolf, involves deep, sometimes painful massage. Intense pressure is applied to various parts of the body. Rolfing practitioners believe that emotional disturbances, physical pain, and other problems can occur when the body is out of alignment—for example, as a result of poor posture. This method takes 10 sessions to complete.

Like the ancient Oriental science of acupuncture, Shiatsu and acupressure are based on the concept of meridians, or invisible channels of flowing energy in the body. The massage therapist presses down on particular points along these channels to release blocked energy and untie knots of muscle tension. For this approach the patient wears loosely fitted clothes, lies on the floor or on a futon, and is not given oil or lotion for the skin.

Trigger point therapy, a neuromuscular technique, focuses in on a painful area, or trigger point, in a muscle. A trigger point might be associated with a problem in another part of the body. Using the fingers or an instrument, such as a rounded piece of wood, concentrated pressure is placed on the irritated area in order to "deactivate" the trigger point.

All of these methods of massage can be altered and intermingled depending on the client's needs. Massage therapists can be proficient in one or many of the methods, and usually tailor a session to the individual.

Requirements

High School

Since massage therapists need to know more than just technical skills, many practitioners use the basic knowledge learned in high school as a foundation to build a solid career in the field. High school students interested in massage therapy should take fundamental science courses, such as chemistry, anatomy, and biology, to prepare them for the health and anatomy classes they will take while completing their certification. English, psychology, and other classes relating to communications and human development will also be useful. If you think you might wish to run your own massage therapy business someday, computer and business courses are essential.

Postsecondary Training

Those who wish to enter the field are advised to attend an accredited massage therapy school. In the United States, there are more than 60 schools accredited or approved by the American Massage Therapy Association (AMTA). Students can begin training for a career in massage therapy directly out of high school. Programs generally last one year. Accredited or approved schools provide at least 500 hours of classroom instruction, of which at least 300 hours are in massage theory and technique, 100 hours in the study of anatomy and physiology, and 100 hours in program-specific coursework. Most programs require students to participate in elective clinics, which allows advanced students the chance to practice their techniques through volunteering massage services to outreach programs such as hospices, hospitals, or shelters. Students can specialize in particular disciplines, such as infant massage or rehabilitative massage. Basic first aid and cardiopulmonary resuscitation (CPR) must also be learned. Other organizations, such as some state medical boards, may require more than 500 hours of instruction. When choosing a school, an applicant should pay close attention to the philosophy and curricula of the program, since a wide range of program options exist.

Certification or Licensing

In about one-fourth of the states, massage therapists must have a license to practice. Requirements may include a written test and a demonstration of massage therapy techniques. Since 1992, the National Certification Board for Therapeutic Massage and Bodywork has offered a certification exam covering massage theory and practice, human anatomy, physiology, kinesiology, business practices, and associated techniques and methods. Legislation is currently being considered to regulate certification across the country.

Other Requirements

Physical requirements of massage therapists generally include the ability to use their hands and other tools to rub or press on the client's body. Manual dexterity is usually required to administer the treatments, as is the ability to stand for at least an hour at a time. Special modifications or accommodations can often be made for persons with different abilities.

A person interested in becoming a massage therapist should be above all nurturing and caring. Constance Bickford, a certified massage therapist in Chicago, thinks that it is necessary to be both flexible and creative: easily adaptable to the needs of the client, as well as able to use different techniques to help the client feel better. Listening well and responding to the client is vital, as is focusing all attention on the task at hand. A massage therapist needs to tune in to the person he or she is working on rather than zone out, thinking about the grocery list or what to cook for supper. An effective massage is a mindful one, where massage therapist and client work together toward improved health.

A massage therapist should also be trustworthy and sensitive. Someone receiving a massage may feel awkward lying naked in an office covered by a sheet, listening to music while a stranger kneads his or her muscles. A good massage therapist will make the client feel comfortable in what could potentially be perceived as a vulnerable situation.

People considering opening up their own business should be prepared for busy and slow times. In order to both serve their clients well and stay in business, they should be adequately staffed during rush seasons, and must be financially able to withstand dry spells.

Exploring

The best way to become familiar with massage therapy is to get a massage. Interested people should make appointments with various types of massage therapists to gain firsthand experience in massage therapy and have the opportunity to talk with therapists about the field.

A less costly approach is to find a book on massage instruction at a local public library or bookstore. Massage techniques can then be practiced at home. Books on self-massage are available. Many books discuss in detail the theoretical basis for the techniques. Videos that demonstrate massage techniques are available as well.

Volunteering at a hospice or shelter can also give students practical experience in caring for others and developing good listening methods. It is important for massage therapists to listen well and respond appropriately to their clients' needs. The massage therapist must make clients feel comfortable, and volunteer work can help foster the skills necessary to achieve this.

Employers

After graduating from an accredited or approved school of massage therapy, there are a number of possibilities for employment. Doctors' offices, hospitals, clinics, health clubs, resorts, country clubs, cruise ships, community service organizations, and nursing homes, for example, all employ massage therapists. Some chiropractors have a massage therapist on staff to whom they can refer patients. Most opportunities for massage therapists will be in larger, urban areas with population growth, although massage therapy is slowly spreading to more rural areas as well.

Starting Out

The American Massage Therapy Association offers job placement information to certified massage therapists who belong to the organization. Massage therapy schools have job placement offices. Newspapers often list jobs. Some graduates are able to enter the field as self-employed massage therapists, scheduling their own appointments and managing their own offices.

Networking is a valuable tool in maintaining a successful massage therapy enterprise. Many massage therapists get clients through referrals, and often rely on word of mouth to build a solid customer base. Beginning massage therapists might wish to consult businesses about arranging onsite massage sessions for their employees.

Health fairs are also good places to distribute information about massage therapy practices and learn about other services in the industry. Often, organizers of large sporting events will employ massage therapists to give massages to athletes at the finish line. These events may include marathons and runs or bike rides done to raise money for charitable organizations.

Advancement

For self-employed massage therapists, advancement is measured by reputation, the ability to draw clients, and the fees charged for services. Health clubs, country clubs, and other institutions have supervisory positions for massage therapists. In a community service organization, massage therapists may be promoted to the position of health service director. Licensed massage therapists often become instructors or advisors at schools for massage therapy. They may also make themselves available to advise individuals or companies on the short- and long-term benefits of massage therapy, and how massage therapy can be introduced into professional work environments.

Earnings

The earnings of massage therapists vary greatly with the level of experience and location of practice. Some entry-level massage therapists earn as little as minimum wage (around $10,712 per year), but with experience, a massage therapist can charge from $10 to $70 for a one-hour session. Assuming 20 hours per week with clients is typical, a highly compensated massage therapist could make $72,800 and up per year. Additional earnings are made from tips. The average rate in the United States for a one-hour session is about $50. Massage therapists are not, however, paid for the time spent on bookkeeping, maintaining their offices, waiting for customers to arrive, and looking for new clients. Those who are self-employed—more than two-thirds of all massage therapists—must also pay a self-employment tax and provide their own benefits. With membership in some national organizations, self-employed massage therapists may be eligible for group life, health, liability, and renter's insurance through the organization's insurance agency.

Massage therapists employed by a health club usually get free or discounted membership to the club. Those who work for resorts or on cruise ships can get free or discounted travel and accommodations, in addition to full access to the club's facilities when not on duty. Massage therapists employed by a sports team often get to attend the team's sporting events.

Work Environment

Massage therapists work in clean, comfortable settings. Because a relaxed environment is essential, the massage room may be dim, and soft music, scents, and oils are often used. Since massage therapists may see a number of people per day, it is important to maintain a hygienic working area. This involves changing sheets on the massage table after each client, as well as cleaning and sterilizing any implements used, and washing hands frequently.

Massage therapists employed by businesses may use a portable massage chair—that is, a padded chair that leaves the client in a forward-leaning position ideal for massage of the back and neck. Some massage therapists work out of their homes or travel to the homes of their clients.

The workweek of a massage therapist is typically 35 to 40 hours, which may include evenings and weekends. On average, fewer than 20 hours per week are spent with clients, and the other hours are spent making appointments and taking care of other business-related details.

Since the physical work is sometimes demanding, massage therapists need to take measures to prevent repetitive stress disorders, such as carpal tunnel syndrome. Also, for their own personal safety, massage therapists who work out of their homes or have odd office hours need to be particularly careful about scheduling appointments with unknown clients.

Outlook

The U.S. Bureau of Labor Statistics does not keep records on the number of massage therapists in the United States. In 1997, however, the industry estimated the number of practitioners to be about 200,000. The employment outlook for massage therapists is good through the year 2006. For a 10-year period beginning in the early 1980s, the AMTA had a tenfold increase in the number of new members and a fourfold increase in the number of accredited or approved schools. The growing acceptance of massage therapy as an important health care discipline has led to the creation of additional jobs for massage therapists in many sectors.

One certified massage therapist points to sports massage as one of the fastest growing specialties in the field. The increasing popularity of professional sports leads to massage therapists becoming key members of a team's staff. This causes a greater public awareness of the physical benefits of massage. She also considers business consulting to be a rapidly increasing enterprise. With the current low rate of unemployment in the United States, employers are trying to encourage good employees to stay in their jobs by offering perks. Employers want their workers to stay healthy, happy, and productive; massage therapy can help them achieve this goal.

For More Information

For more information about massage therapy, contact:

American Massage Therapy Association (AMTA)
820 Davis Street, Suite 100
Evanston, IL 60201-4444
Tel: 847-864-0123
Web: http://www.amtamassage.org/

Associated Bodywork and Massage Professionals
28677 Buffalo Park Road
Evergreen, CO 80439-7347
Tel: 800-458-2267
Web: http://www.abmp.com/

For information about certification and education requirements for the state in which you plan to work, contact:

National Certification Board for Therapeutic Massage and Bodywork
8201 Greensboro Drive, Suite 300
McLean, VA 22102
Tel: 800-296-0664 or 703-610-9015
Web: http://www.ncbtmb.com/

Naturopaths

School Subjects
- Biology
- Business
- Chemistry

Personal Skills
- Helping/teaching
- Technical/scientific

Work Environment
- Primarily indoors
- Primarily one location

Minimum Education Level
- Medical degree

Salary Range
- $35,000 to $80,000 to $100,000

Certification or Licensing
- Required by certain states

Outlook
- Faster than the average

Overview

Naturopaths—also called *naturopathic physicians*—are licensed health professionals who practice an approach to health care called *naturopathic medicine*. Naturopathic medicine (also called naturopathy) is a distinct system of health care that uses a variety of natural approaches to health and healing, including clinical nutrition, counseling, herbal medicine, homeopathy, and physical therapy. Naturopaths (pronounced "nature-o-paths") recognize the integrity of the whole person, and they emphasize the individual's inherent capacity for self-healing.

History

The therapies and philosophy on which naturopathic medicine is based can be traced back to the ancient healing arts of early civilizations. Healers in ancient times used natural treatments that relied on the body's innate ability to heal itself. They made use of foods, herbs, water, massage, and fasting.

Hippocrates, who is thought by many to be the father of modern medicine, is also often considered to be the earliest predecessor of naturopathic physicians. He used many natural approaches to health care. He is reported to have told his followers, "Let your food be your medicine and your medicine be your food."

During the 18th and 19th centuries, an alternative healing movement in Europe contributed to the development of naturopathic medicine. The German homeopathic practitioner John H. Scheel is credited with first using the term "naturopath" in 1895.

Dr. Benedict Lust introduced naturopathy to the United States. He founded the American School of Naturopathy, which graduated its first class in 1902. In 1909, California became the first state to legally regulate the practice of naturopathy. Early naturopaths, Dr. John Kellogg, his brother Will Kellogg, and C. W. Post, helped popularize naturopathy.

Naturopathy flourished in the early part of the 20th century. By 1930, there were more than 20 naturopathic schools and 10,000 practitioners nationwide. With the rise of modern pharmaceuticals and allopathic (conventional) medicine, naturopathic medicine experienced a decline during the 1940s and 1950s. In the last three decades of the 20th century, however, due to the rapidly growing public interest in alternative health care approaches, naturopathic medicine experienced a strong revival.

According to the National Institutes of Health, around 1,000 licensed naturopathic doctors (NDs) were practicing in the United States in 1993. By 1998, there were about 1,700 practicing NDs and 1,500 students training to become naturopathic physicians.

The Job

In North America, 12 states, four provinces, and Puerto Rico license naturopathic doctors. In these areas, NDs provide complete diagnostic and therapeutic services. They are consulted as primary care physicians, and they receive referrals from other physicians. Patients consult naturopaths for a variety of health problems, including digestive disorders, chronic fatigue, asthma, depression, infections, obesity, colds, and flu.

When seeing a new patient, NDs first take a careful medical history to understand the state of health of the whole individual—body, mind, and spirit. They consider the patient as a whole person who has something out of balance, and they don't just focus on the symptoms of illness. Naturopathic doctors ask many questions about lifestyle, eating habits, stress, and many other issues. They listen carefully to determine what imbalance may be causing illness or preventing recovery. They may spend an hour to an hour and a half with a new patient.

Naturopathic physicians take a holistic approach to health care. They recognize the connection between the health of the mind and the health of the body. Depression, stress, and fear all can have an impact on physical health. Naturopaths listen carefully to their patients to learn about the impact of outside forces, such as a stressful work environment or family situation, that may be contributing to the illness.

Once they make a diagnosis, NDs prescribe a course of treatment. Naturopathic physicians practice health care that supports the body's self-healing processes. They recognize that the human body has a natural capability to heal itself, so they use methods of care that will work with these processes. Naturopathic doctors use many natural and noninvasive healing techniques. They are trained in counseling, herbal medicine, clinical nutrition, homeopathy, hydrotherapy, massage, and other types of physical medicine.

Naturopathic physicians believe that most conventional doctors treat only the illness, not the patient. In treating the patient, NDs recommend methods that have more lasting effects. They recommend changes in diet, prescribe botanical medicine (herbs), and recommend vitamins. They may even offer counseling to help the patient make lifestyle changes.

Naturopathic medicine is most effective in treating chronic illness. Like many other alternative health care approaches, naturopathy is not usually used for acute, life-threatening illnesses. Some NDs are trained in techniques of minor surgery. They do not perform major surgery, but they may be involved in the recovery process after surgery. For some conditions, naturopaths may refer a patient to a specialist, such as a cardiologist or oncologist. Even while a patient is seeing a specialist, the naturopath continues to work with the individual and the self-healing process. This can result in a team-care approach.

Although naturopathic physicians are currently licensed by only 12 states, licensed NDs practice in every state. (Doctors licensed by the state of Arizona, for example, can maintain their licenses even if they practice in another state.) However, NDs who practice in states that do not offer licensing must restrict the scope of their practices to areas such as homeopathy (a form of therapy that emphasizes natural remedies and treatments) and nutrition counseling.

The majority of naturopaths are in private practice. That means that they must have the skills to run a business on a day-to-day basis. They interview, hire, and train staff and oversee the functioning of an office. More and more insurance companies are covering naturopathic medicine in states that offer licenses, and NDs must be able to oversee complicated insurance billing procedures in order to be paid for their services.

Requirements

High School

If you want to pursue a career in naturopathy, you'll be entering a premed program in college, so you'll want to take high school science courses, such as biology and chemistry. The physical education courses of some high schools offer instruction in health, nutrition, and exercise that would help prepare you for important aspects of work as a naturopath.

English, psychology, and sociology courses are valuable in helping you sharpen your communication and people skills. As a naturopath, you will need to be an excellent listener and communicator. Much of a naturopathic physician's work involves listening to and counseling clients. Business, math, and computer classes are important to prepare you for running a business.

Postsecondary Training

A student of naturopathic medicine must first complete a premed undergraduate program before pursuing a Doctor of Naturopathic Medicine degree (ND or sometimes NMD). Courses in chemistry and other basic medical sciences are required. Courses in nutrition and psychology are also important. You should contact the accredited naturopathic colleges as early as possible in order to ensure that you complete the courses required by the school of your choice.

When you're searching for a naturopathic medical school, find one that's accredited and offers the Doctor of Naturopathic Medicine degree. Schools without accreditation offer correspondence courses and may offer certificates. Only a degree from an accredited school will prepare you to become a licensed naturopath. The professional associations listed at the end of this article can help you learn about accredited schools and their requirements.

The naturopathic doctoral degree is a four-year program requiring courses in anatomy, physiology, biochemistry, and other basic medical sciences. Students must also take courses in nutrition, botanical medicine, homeopathy, naturopathic obstetrics, psychological medicine, and minor surgery. In addition to course instruction, students receive extensive clinical training.

Certification or Licensing

To practice medicine as a naturopathic physician, you must be licensed in the state in which you practice. Licensing is available in 12 states: Alaska, Arizona, Connecticut, Florida, Hawaii, Maine, Montana, New Hampshire, Oregon, Utah, Vermont, and Washington. All state licenses are contingent upon passing the Naturopathic Physicians Licensing Examinations (NPLEX), a standardized test for all naturopathic physicians in North America. As this field of health care continues to gain wide acceptance, the number of licensed states is expected to grow. To maintain a license in naturopathic medicine, NDs are required to take 30 hours of continuing education courses every two years.

Naturopathic physicians who practice in unlicensed states are not allowed to practice as physicians. They can still use their skills and knowledge to help people improve their lives, but they usually limit their practices to homeopathy or nutritional counseling.

Other Requirements

A primary requirement for a successful naturopath is a strong desire to help people improve their lives. You must also have a fundamental belief in the whole-person approach to healing. Because counseling plays such an important role in treatment, naturopathic physicians need excellent listening and communication skills. Keen powers of observation and good decision-making abilities are essential to accurate medical assessment. Like other medical professions, naturopathy requires a commitment to lifelong learning. Idealism and a firm belief in the efficacy of natural approaches to medicine are important. You must have the courage of your convictions and be willing to stand up for your beliefs. Naturopathy has become much more respected within the medical profession in recent years, but it is still unaccepted by some conventional doctors.

Exploring

Contact the professional associations listed at the end of this article for information. Check out the Web site of the International Naturopathic Students' Association (INSA), and take advantage of the opportunity to network with students from all of the naturopathic schools in North America. The Internet has a wealth of information. Some Web sites have chat groups; others have searchable databases.

Make an appointment for a medical checkup with a naturopathic physician. Find out what the practice of naturopathy is like, and think about whether you would like to practice medicine this way. Ask a naturopath to talk with you about the field. Perhaps that person will be willing to be a mentor for you.

Visit the naturopathic colleges that interest you. Sit in on classes. Talk to students about their experiences. Find out what they like and what they don't like. Talk to the faculty and learn about their approaches to teaching. Ask what they see as the best opportunities in the field.

Employers

Most naturopaths go into private or group practice. A few NDs find positions in natural health clinics. Due to the small number of accredited doctoral programs, only a very small percentage of naturopaths become teachers. The federal government is encouraging research into the efficacy of alternative health care approaches. More research opportunities are becoming available, and an increasing number of naturopaths are pursuing this aspect of the profession. The thriving natural food industry is providing more opportunities for naturopaths as consultants. The majority of NDs work in the 12 states that license them; however, naturopathic physicians can be found throughout the United States.

Starting Out

The placement office of the naturopathic college you attend can help you in searching for that first job. Join professional organizations, attend meetings, and get to know people in your field. Networking is one of the most powerful ways of finding a new position. Get to know professionals in other areas of alternative health care. As other alternative health care modalities expand, they will be more likely to include naturopaths in alternative clinics.

As a newly licensed naturopathic physician, you might begin working on a salary or income-sharing basis in a clinic or in an established practice with another naturopath or other health care professional. This would allow you to start practicing without the major financial investment of equipping an office. You might be able to purchase the practice of an ND who is retiring or moving. This is usually easier than starting a new solo practice because the practice will already have patients. However, some newly licensed practitioners do start immediately in private practice.

Advancement

Because most naturopaths work in private or group practice, advancement frequently depends on the physician's dedication to building a patient base. As an ND in private practice, you will need a general sense of how to run a successful business. You must promote your practice within the community and develop a network of contacts with conventional medical doctors or other alternative practitioners who may refer patients to you.

Some naturopaths advance by starting their own clinics with other naturopaths or with other alternative health practitioners. In any medical field, learning is lifelong, and many naturopaths derive a sense of professional satisfaction from keeping up on changes in allopathic medicine and in natural health research. A few very experienced NDs write textbooks or become professors at the accredited universities. With the growing government interest in research into natural health care, more naturopathic physicians will find opportunities for advancement as researchers.

Earnings

Most naturopaths can make a comfortable living in private practice, but naturopathic medicine is generally not as financially rewarding as some other branches of medicine. Financial success as a naturopath requires dedication to building up a practice and promoting natural health treatment. Although a well-established naturopath can make up to $200,000 a year, most earn much less. A beginning naturopath earns around $35,000 a year. After some years of practice, NDs generally average $80,000 to $100,000 per year.

Income depends on such factors as the size and geographic location of practices. In states that license NDs, the population is typically more interested in natural health. In those states, naturopaths may have larger practices than in states that do not license.

Since most naturopathic physicians are in private practice, they must provide their own benefits. Those who work in clinics, universities, or research may receive benefits, such as vacation and sick pay, insurance, and contributions to retirement accounts.

Work Environment

Naturopathic physicians work in clean, quiet, comfortable offices. Most solo practitioners and group practices have an office suite. The suite generally has a reception area. In clinics, several professionals may share this area. The suite also contains examining rooms and treatment rooms. In a clinic where several professionals work, there sometimes are separate offices for the individual professionals. Many naturopaths have an assistant or office staff. Those who are in private practices or partnerships need to have good business skills and self-discipline to be successful.

Naturopaths who work in clinics, research settings, or universities need to work well in a group environment. They frequently work under supervision or in a team with other professionals. They may have offices of their own or they may share offices with team members, depending on the facility. In these organizations, the physical work environment varies, but it will generally be clean and comfortable. Because they are larger, these settings may be noisier than the smaller practices.

Most naturopathic physicians work about 42 hours per week, although many put in longer hours. Larger organizations may determine the hours of work, but NDs in private practice can set their own. Evening and weekend hours are sometimes scheduled to accommodate patients' needs.

Outlook

Naturopathic medicine gained much wider acceptance in the late 1990s. Trends were very promising. Three states added licensing requirements, bringing the total number of licensing states to 12. The first naturopathic college within a university was opened at the University of Bridgeport in Connecticut.

Public interest in alternative health care is growing. Many health-conscious individuals are attracted to naturopathy because of its natural, holistic, preventive approach. The average life span is increasing. As a result, the number of older people is also increasing. The elderly frequently have more health care needs, and the growth of this segment of the population will increase the demand for NDs.

An encouraging development is that more insurance policies are beginning to cover alternative health care services. This still varies according to the insurer, but in states where NDs are licensed, more companies cover their services.

The demand for naturopathic physicians is expected to grow faster than the average for other careers into the early 21st century. According to Robert Lofft, executive director of the Council on Naturopathic Medical Education, "NDs are in great demand. Many cannot accept any more patients. The demand is outpacing the supply." While the demand for naturopathy is increasing, college enrollments are also growing. New NDs may find increasing competition in geographic areas where other practitioners are already located.

For More Information

For information about naturopathic medicine, accredited schools, and state licensing status, contact:

American Association of Naturopathic Physicians
601 Valley Street, Suite 105
Seattle, WA 98109
Tel: 206-298-0126
Web: http://www.naturopathic.org

For an opportunity to network with students from naturopathic medical schools in North America, visit their attractive, informative Web site:

International Naturopathic Students' Association (INSA)
Web: http://www.members.tripod.com/~INSA/index.html

Nutritionists

Biology Chemistry Health	School Subjects
Helping/teaching Technical/scientific	Personal Skills
Primarily indoors Primarily one location	Work Environment
Associate's degree	Minimum Education Level
$20,000 to $35,000 to $70,000+	Salary Range
Recommended	Certification or Licensing
About as fast as the average	Outlook

Overview

Nutritionists seek to provide the people for whom they are responsible with foods that will improve or maintain their health. Nutritionists work for themselves or for institutions of various kinds, such as hospitals, schools, restaurants, and hotels—any place where food is served or nutritional counseling is required. A hospital nutritionist, for example, will both ensure that the food served in the cafeteria is nourishing and create special diets for patients with particular nutritional problems and needs.

History

Nutrition has been an important concern to people throughout the world for millennia, and the use of food as medicine has been recognized throughout recorded history. In India, the form of medicine known as Ayurveda has used diets tailored to individuals to cure or to maintain health for as long as five thousand years. Traditional Chinese medicine (TCM), which is approximately as old as Ayurveda, makes use of many dietary recommendations and pro-scriptions. Both forms of medicine are still widely used in their countries of origin, and both have spread to other parts of the world.

In ancient Greece, philosophers and healers noted the connection between diet and health, and ultimately it was the Greek practice of careful observation and research that gave rise to the scientific method, on which the modern Western approach to nutrition is based. It should be understood, however, that observation and research were also important parts of virtual-ly all other medical traditions.

A major breakthrough in nutrition occurred in the 18th century, when the French chemist Antoine-Laurent Lavoisier began to study the way the body uses food energy, or calories. He also examined the relationship between heat production and the use of energy, and his work has caused him to be known as the "father of nutrition."

By the early 20th century, vitamins had been studied, and the relation-ship between certain diets and certain illnesses came to be understood. By 1940, most vitamins and minerals had been discovered and studied, and the field of nutrition had made tremendous strides. Since that time, advances in technology have enabled scientists to learn far more about nutrition than was possible earlier. At present, much is known, but much remains to be learned. It often happens that one study contradicts another regarding the benefits or dangers of certain foods, as anyone who reads a newspaper knows.

The Job

Nutritionists can be divided into two primary groups: nutritionists and *dieti-tians*. The difference between the two is that dietitians usually have more comprehensive training than other nutritionists do. There are no specific requirements for nutritionists, and theoretically anyone could set up shop as a nutritionist with little or no training. In reality, however, most nutritionists have at least two years of college-level training in nutrition, and many nutri-tionists have advanced degrees. If they did not have sufficient training, they would be unlikely to be financially successful.

In the United States, only nutritionists who have completed the exten-sive training and testing approved by the American Dietetic Association (ADA) and have thereby earned the designation Registered Dietitian (RD) can be called dietitians. There is, however, another designation for registered dietetic professionals: Dietetic Technician, Registered (DTR).

For the most part, those who hold prestigious positions in institutions are dietitians. Many positions require that an applicant be a DTR or an RD. Many nutritionists in private practice, however, do not have—and do not need—either of these designations. For the rest of this article, except where specific differences are pointed out, the terms *nutritionist* and *dietitian* will be used interchangeably.

There are many specialties within the field of nutrition, and the field is changing rapidly. One reason for this change is that the public has become more aware of the importance of nutrition in recent years, and this development has opened up new areas for nutritionists. The descriptions of nutritional specialties that follow are by no means complete.

Clinical dietitians are in charge of planning and supervising the preparation of diets designed for specific patients, and they work for such institutions as hospitals and retirement homes. In many cases, their patients cannot eat certain foods for medical reasons, such as diabetes or liver failure, and the dietitians must see that these patients receive nourishing meals. Clinical dietitians work closely with doctors, who advise them regarding the patients' health and the foods that the patients cannot eat. It is often part of a clinical dietitian's job to educate patients about nutritional principles.

The job of the *community dietitian* usually involves working for a clinic, government health program, social service agency, or similar organization. These dietitians may counsel individuals or advise the members of certain groups—such as the elderly, families, and pregnant women—regarding nutritional problems, proper eating, and sensible grocery shopping.

Although most nutritionists do some kind of teaching in the course of their work, *teaching dietitians* specialize in education. They usually work for hospitals, and they may teach full time or part time. Sometimes teaching dietitians also perform other tasks, such as running a food-service operation, especially in small colleges. In larger institutions, however, those tasks are generally performed by different people. In some cases, teaching dietitians also perform research.

There are many kinds of *consultant dietitians,* who work for such organizations as schools, restaurants, grocery store chains, manufacturers of food-service equipment, pharmaceutical companies, and private companies of various kinds. Some of these organizations have home economics departments that need the services of nutritionists. Some consultants spend much of their time advising individuals rather than organizations. One lucrative area for consultants is working with athletes and sports teams, helping to maximize athletes' performance and extend the length of their careers.

Administrative dietitians are managers, and they must not only have good people skills but also must be effective project managers. They run food-service operations, work in restaurant management, and direct other kinds of nutrition-related operations. Among their duties are creating budgets, drawing up work policies, and enforcing institutional and government regulations that relate to safety and sanitation.

Research dietitians typically work for government organizations, universities, hospitals, pharmaceutical companies, and manufacturers, and they may specialize in any of a vast number of research subjects. They may conduct research themselves or manage those who do. Research dietitians often seek to improve existing food products or to find alternatives to foods that are unhealthy when eaten in substantial portions.

Requirements

High School

If you want to be a nutritionist, you should take as many courses as possible in health, biology, chemistry, and mathematics. Students who are not sufficiently prepared in high school are likely to struggle with college courses in mathematics, biochemistry, and so forth. Communication skills are also important, since nutritionists must interact effectively with clients, employers, and colleagues. Even researchers who spend most of their time in the lab must cooperate with colleagues and write clear, accurate reports on the results of their work. For this reason, a nutritionist must be well versed in spoken and written English. Be sure to study family and consumer science. It also is a good idea to take a course in psychology, which generally is taught in college nutrition programs and is an important aspect of the work of many nutritionists. At the same time, doing as much reading as possible about nutrition, health, anatomy, and so forth is essential. If some important subjects are not taught in your high school, study them on your own.

Postsecondary Training

The kind of postsecondary training you need has everything to do with the area of nutrition in which you want to work. If you want to work in a major institution, you should become an RD or a DTR. To do that, you will need to fulfill the requirements of the ADA: attend an accredited college or university (the degree may be in dietetics, food service, or another related area), complete a practice program, take and pass a registration examination, and take required continuing-education courses. If you want to teach, do research, or work in public health, you should get a bachelor's degree and one or more advanced degrees. In that situation, it may be a good idea both to become an RD and to obtain one or more postgraduate degrees. In such a case, you might want to get a master's degree from an institution that offers the practice program required for certification as an RD.

Certification or Licensing

To become an RD, a person must have at least a bachelor's degree from an accredited college or university and must take courses approved by the Commission on Accreditation/Approval for Dietetics Education (CAADE), which is a division of the ADA. In addition, he or she must complete a supervised practice program authorized by the CAADE. Such programs, which usually take six to twelve months to complete, can be taken at food-service organizations, health care facilities, or authorized colleges or universities. In many cases, students choose to complete master's programs that include a practice program. After completing these requirements, the student must pass a comprehensive examination given by the Commission on Dietetic Registration (CDR). After that, the new RD must complete continuing-education requirements to stay registered.

To become a DTR, a student must complete at least a two-year associate's degree at an accredited college or university, complete an approved DTR program that includes at least 450 hours of supervised practice, pass an exam, and complete continuing-education requirements in order to stay registered.

Registration as an RD or a DTR is not invariably necessary for nutritionists, but it is a good idea for many in the profession. In the United States, 40 states have laws relating to dietetics, 12 states require certification, 27 require licensing, and 1 requires registration. Many positions are open only to those who are registered.

Other Requirements

Because there are so many technical requirements in the field of nutrition, nutritionists must be detail oriented and able to think analytically. Math and science are a major part of both training and work. Nutritionists must be comfortable making decisions and acting on them. Even those who do not work as consultants have to be disciplined and decisive.

For most nutritionists, flexibility is crucial. Karen Petty, RD, an administrator who began her career as a clinical dietitian, says about working in institutional food service: "You will never be able to please everyone, because everyone has different tastes in food. You learn to be able to take criticism and go on to try to please the majority."

People who want to become administrators must have people skills. On that subject, Petty says: "When I'm asked what is the hardest part of my job, I never hesitate to say it's personnel management." For administrators, the ability to communicate clearly and effectively is particularly important.

Exploring

One of the best ways to learn about nutrition is to get a job in a food-related business such as a restaurant or a hospital cafeteria. There is no substitute for observing and interacting with nutritionists. Another approach is to contact nutritionists and ask them about their work. You should also learn to cook. If you are going to be in the food business, you should know how to prepare healthy and attractive meals.

Employers

Many kinds of government and private organizations hire nutritionists, and the kinds of available opportunities continue to increase. There are opportunities in hospitals, schools of all levels, community health programs, day care centers, correctional facilities, health clubs, weight-management clinics, health-maintenance organizations (HMOs), nursing homes, government organizations, food-service companies, food equipment manufacturers, sports teams, pharmaceutical companies, and grocery store chains. Among the large organizations that need nutritionists are the armed forces, which have to feed their personnel as well and as cheaply as possible.

Starting Out

Because most nutritionists are extensively trained and usually have some practical experience before they look for their first job, they tend to know in which kinds of organizations they want to work. Most colleges and universities provide placement services, and people often find work through connections they make at school or in practice programs. For this reason, it is wise to make as many professional connections as possible.

Some parts of the country have more nutritionists than others, and beginning nutritionists should consider taking positions out of their areas in order to get started in the business. Jobs can be found via trade journals, national and state conventions, Web sites, classified ads, and specialized employment agencies. Although it is possible to call organizations to learn about job opportunities, the most effective way to find work is through personal contacts.

Advancement

There are various ways to advance in the business. One of the best is further education. A nutritionist with an associate's degree may go on to become a DTR or an RD. A DTR can advance by becoming an RD. Nutritionists who have only a bachelor's degree will have more opportunities if they obtain an RD designation. Those who are already RDs may wish to obtain advanced degrees, which will enable them to apply for research, teaching, or public health positions that are not otherwise open to them.

In the field of nutrition, as in most others, seniority, reliability, expertise, and experience count. An experienced clinical dietitian might ultimately become an administrative dietitian, for example, and a research dietitian might wind up in charge of a research department.

Earnings

In 1997, according to the ADA, 45 percent of entry-level RDs made between $25,000 and $35,000 a year, while 32 percent made between $35,000 and $45,000. Many experienced RDs made more than $50,000 yearly, and some of them made $70,000 or more. In the same year, 63 percent of DTRs who had been working no longer than five years made between $20,001 and $30,000, while 15 percent made between $30,001 and $40,000. It is reasonable to conclude that other nutritionists made salaries that fall in roughly the same range. One important factor is location. A dietitian in Los Angeles, California, for example, is likely to make (and need) more money than a dietitian in Boise, Idaho.

Work Environment

Nutritionists generally work in offices or kitchens. Such environments are usually clean, well lit, and effectively illuminated, although some kitchens may be hot and stifling. Some nutritionists sit much of the time, while others spend all day on their feet. Most work 40-hour weeks, but some—especially those who work for hospitals and restaurants—are required to work on weekends and at odd hours. Part-time positions are also common.

Some hospitals offer nutritionists room, board, and laundry services for a nominal fee, but this arrangement is becoming less common. In the past, many college dietitians lived in apartments provided by the school, but this arrangement is also becoming a thing of the past, except where nutritionists run food-service operations in residence halls.

Benefits such as health insurance, sick pay, vacations, and 401(k) plans are as prevalent in the field of nutrition as they are in other fields. Naturally, nutritionists who run their own businesses must make their own arrangements in these areas.

Outlook

According to the U.S. Department of Labor's 1998-99 *Occupational Outlook Handbook* (OOH), employment of dietitians and nutritionists will grow about as fast as the average for all occupations through 2006. One contributor to the continued growth is increasing awareness of the importance of nutrition. People who would not have consulted nutritionists in years past will do so now. Another contributor is the fact that the population is aging rapidly, which will bring about an increased need for nutritional counseling and planning in nursing homes, home health care agencies, community health programs, and prisons. Additionally, there will be a need to replace aging nutritionists and dietitians. One area that will experience decreased demand, says the OOH, is that of hospitals. Inpatient treatment is expected to decline, while outpatient treatment will increase. Many hospitals are expected to hire contractors to handle food-service operations.

For More Information

The ADA is the single best source of information about careers in dietetics. Its Web site is an excellent resource that provides detailed information and links to other organizations and resources.

American Dietetic Association
216 West Jackson Boulevard, Suite 800
Chicago, IL 60606
Tel: 800-877-1600, ext. 4897
Web: http://www.eatright.org

The goal of the ASNS is to improve people's quality of life through the nutritional sciences. It is a good source of educational and career information.

American Society for Nutritional Sciences
9650 Rockville Pike
Bethesda, MD 20814
Tel: 301-530-7050
Web: http://www.faseb.org/asns

Oriental Medicine Practitioners

Biology Psychology	School Subjects
Helping/teaching Technical/scientific	Personal Skills
Primarily indoors Primarily one location	Work Environment
Associate's degree	Minimum Education Level
$10,700 to $40,000 to $100,000	Salary Range
Required by certain states	Certification or Licensing
Faster than the average	Outlook

Overview

Oriental medicine practitioners are health care professionals who practice a variety of health care therapies that are part of the ancient healing system of Oriental medicine. *Oriental medicine* is a comprehensive system of health care. It includes several major modalities: acupuncture, Chinese herbology, Oriental bodywork or massage (tuina), exercise (qigong), and dietary therapy. Each of these major areas has numerous variations, but all forms are based on traditional Oriental medicine principles. An Oriental medicine practitioner may practice one or many of the therapies of Oriental medicine.

Over one-third of the world's population relies on Oriental medicine practitioners for the enhancement of health and for prevention and treatment of disease. In the West, Oriental medicine is rapidly growing in popularity as an alternative health care system. In 1998, there were approximately 10,000 Oriental medicine/acupuncture practitioners in the United States. There were around 1,400 members of the American Oriental Bodywork Therapy Association.

History

Traditional Chinese medicine (TCM) has over 3,000 years of clinical history. The basic principles of TCM were first recorded in the Yellow Emperor's *Classic of Internal Medicine (Huang Di Nei Ching)* in China around 2,300 years ago. Traditional Chinese medicine practitioners continually applied, developed, and refined those principles for centuries.

Oriental medicine is based on an energetic model of health that is fundamentally different from the biochemical model of Western medicine. The ancient Chinese recognized a vital energy that they believed to be the animating force behind all life. They called this life force *qi* (or *chi*, both pronounced "chee"). They discovered that the body's qi flows along specific channels—called *meridians*—in the body. Each meridian is related to a particular physiological system and internal organ. When the body's qi is unbalanced, or when the flow of qi along the channels is blocked or disrupted, disease, pain, and other physical and emotional conditions result. The fundamental purpose of all forms of Oriental medicine is to restore and maintain balance in the body's qi.

As traditional Chinese medicine spread gradually throughout Southeast Asia, each culture adapted the principles of TCM to its own healing methods. The Japanese, Koreans, and other Asian peoples contributed to the development of the ancient Chinese principles and developed their own variations based upon those principles. In recognition of the contributions of many Asian cultures, TCM is now referred to as traditional Oriental medicine (TOM), or simply Oriental medicine (OM).

Since the advent of quantum physics, the Western world has developed a new interest in and appreciation for the bioenergetic model of health of the Oriental world. Western physics is generating a new science of resonance and energy fields that proposes that a person is more a "resonating field" than a substance. Oriental medicine is completely consistent with this "new" concept.

Oriental medicine practitioners are increasingly consulted in Europe, North America, and Russia for general maintenance of health, treatment of disease, and relief of pain. Since the 1970s, acupuncture and Oriental medicine have been among the fastest growing forms of health care in the United States. During the last decade of the 20th century, the increasing interest in alternative medicine in the United States and throughout the world brought Oriental medicine practitioners to the forefront of the field of alternative health care.

The Job

Oriental medicine practitioners usually specialize in one or more of the healing modalities that make up Oriental medicine. In the United States, the educational career paths for Oriental medicine practitioners are currently organized around acupuncture, Oriental medicine (acupuncture and Chinese herbology), and Oriental bodywork, according to Barbara Mitchell, executive director of the National Acupuncture and Oriental Medicine Alliance. She noted that not all disciplines are licensed or recognized in every state. Whatever their specialties may be, they use common approaches to the practice of OM. All therapies are based upon the fundamental principle of diagnosing and seeking to balance disturbances of qi.

Oriental medicine practitioners begin a new relationship with a client by taking a careful history. Next, they use the traditional Chinese approach called the "four examinations" for evaluation and diagnosis. These include asking questions, looking, listening/smelling, and touching. Oriental medicine practitioners use the four examinations to identify signs and symptoms. They synthesize all they learn about the individual into a vivid profile of the whole person—mind, body, and spirit. The first appointment generally requires an hour or more.

The process of examination tells Oriental medicine practitioners what type of disharmony the individual has. The results of the evaluation and diagnosis determine the therapies the practitioner chooses. Depending on their own training and on the needs of the individual client, the Oriental medicine practitioners may recommend one or more of the major modalities: acupuncture, Chinese herbology, Oriental bodywork, exercise, or dietary therapy.

In the West, acupuncture is the best-known form of traditional Oriental medicine, and it is sometimes considered synonymous with Oriental medicine. Acupuncture is a complete medical system that encourages the body to improve functioning and promote natural healing. *Acupuncturists* help their clients maintain good health, and they also treat symptoms and disorders. They insert very thin needles into precise acupuncture points on the skin. They stimulate the acupuncture points to balance the circulation of energy. This influences the health of the whole person. For more detailed information, see the article on acupuncturists.

In the United States, most of the modalities of traditional Chinese medicine are now frequently considered under the more general term of Oriental medicine. However, even practitioners from Japan, Korea, and other Asian countries still consider Chinese herbology to be uniquely Chinese. Chinese herbology (also known as the Chinese herbal sciences) studies the properties of herbs, their energetics, and their therapeutic qualities. It has a 2,000-year history as a distinct body of knowledge—independent of acupuncture. *Chinese herbalists* practice herbal science according to the principals of Oriental medicine. After performing a careful evaluation and diagnosis, they consider all of a person's characteristics to determine which herbs to use in a strategy for restoring the balance of the individual's qi. Chinese herbalists develop herbal formulas based upon the unique combination of the individual's characteristics, symptoms, and primary complaints.

Tuina (or Tui Na—both pronounced "twee nah") is a form of Oriental bodywork or massage that has been used in China for 2,000 years. It is sometimes referred to as Oriental physical therapy. *Tuina practitioners* seek to establish a more harmonious flow of qi through the channels (meridians) of the body. They accomplish this through a variety of different systems: massage, acupressure ("one finger pushing"), energy generation exercises, and manipulation. The tuina practitioner evaluates the individual's specific problems and develops a treatment plan that emphasizes acupressure points and energy meridians as well as pain sites, muscles, and joints. Unlike traditional Western types of massage that involve a more generalized treatment, tuina focuses on specific problem areas. Treatments usually last half an hour to an hour. The number of sessions depends on the needs of the client. Some Oriental bodywork practitioners use Chinese herbs to assist the healing process.

Qigong (sometimes Qi Gong or Chi Kung—all pronounced "chee goong") is a Chinese system of exercise, philosophy, and health care. It is a healing art that combines movement and meditation. The Chinese character "qi" means life force; the character "gong" means to cultivate or engage in. Qigong literally means to cultivate one's life force or vital energy (or in Western terms, resonating bioelectrical field). Qigong has five major traditions: Taoist, Buddhist, Confucian, martial arts, and medical. It has more than a thousand forms. Kung fu is an example of a martial arts qigong. T'ai qi (t'ai chi) has Taoist, martial arts, and self-healing forms. Medical qigong combines meditation with breathing exercises. Through the regular practice of qigong, the circulation of the qi is stimulated. This can help body functions return to normal for those who are sick; it can increase the sense of well-being for those who are already healthy.

Oriental dietary therapy helps to restore harmony to the qi through balancing what the individual eats. When the diet becomes unbalanced, it can trigger disharmony. The Oriental medicine practitioner recommends adjustments in the diet that will restore balance. The therapeutic basis for dietary therapy is the same as for Chinese herbology. The practitioner considers the energetics and therapeutic qualities of each kind of food in order to select precisely the right foods to restore balance to the individual's qi.

In addition to working to help their clients achieve a more balanced state, Oriental medicine practitioners usually have many other duties. Most are self-employed, so they have all of the obligations of running their own businesses. They must keep records of their clients' histories and progress. They have to manage their own client billing. If their services are covered by insurance, they bill the insurance companies. They work to build their clientele. A career in Oriental medicine requires lifelong learning, and practitioners continually study and increase their knowledge of their field.

Requirements

High School

To prepare yourself for a career as an Oriental medicine practitioner, you need to learn to understand the human body, mind, and spirit. Courses in science—particularly biology—will help you prepare for the medical courses ahead. Psychology, philosophy, sociology, and comparative religion classes can help you learn about the mind and spirit. Physical education and sports training will help you prepare for the exercise and massage aspects of Oriental medicine. English, drama, debate, and speech can help you develop the communication skills you will need to relate to your clients and to build your business. Most Oriental medicine practitioners are self-employed, so you will also need business, math, and computer skills.

Postsecondary Training

In the United States, there are presently two defined career paths for Oriental medicine practitioners: acupuncture and Oriental bodywork. More than 60 schools in the United States have courses in Oriental medicine and acupuncture. Most offer master's level programs. For admission to a master's level program in Oriental medicine, virtually every school requires two years of undergraduate study. Others require a bachelor's degree in a related field, such as science, nursing, or premed. Most Oriental medicine programs provide a thorough education in Western sciences as well as Chinese herbology, acupuncture techniques, and all aspects of traditional Oriental medicine.

Choosing a school for Oriental medicine can be complex. An important consideration is where you want to live and practice. State requirements to practice Oriental medicine vary, so be sure the school you choose will prepare you to practice where you want to live.

If you need federal financial assistance, be sure to choose a college that is accredited by the Accreditation Commission for Acupuncture and Oriental Medicine (ACAOM), because the U.S. Department of Education recognizes only programs accredited by ACAOM.

The second career path for Oriental medicine practitioners is the study of tuina—Oriental bodywork therapy. Tuina is not taught as a separate discipline in schools of Oriental medicine. To become an Oriental bodywork therapist, you must first meet the requirements of your state to become a massage therapist.

Most massage therapy schools require a high school diploma for entrance. Postsecondary or previous study of science, psychology, and business can be helpful. Some schools require a personal interview. You should look for an accredited massage school that offers a minimum of 500 hours of training. The training should include anatomy, physiology, kinesiology (the principles of mechanics and anatomy as they relate to human movement), ethics, and business practices. In addition, the school should provide courses in the theory and practice of massage therapy and supervised hands-on training. For an in-depth discussion of massage therapy, be sure to see the article on massage therapists.

Once you have completed your program in general massage therapy, you can specialize in Oriental bodywork therapy. Some massage schools offer courses in Oriental bodywork. A specialty in Oriental bodywork requires 150 to 500 hours of additional training. The American Oriental Bodywork Therapy Association (AOBTA) can supply you with information about schools that offer training in tuina.

Certification or Licensing

The National Certification Commission for Acupuncture and Oriental Medicine (NCCAOM) certifies acupuncturists and promotes nationally recognized standards for acupuncture and Oriental medicine. In order to qualify to take the NCCAOM exam, you must complete a three-year accredited master's level or candidate program. You must complete this three-year program at a school accredited by the Accreditation Commission for Acupuncture and Oriental Medicine (ACAOM) or through a master's level program.

Licensing is a requirement established by a government body (in this case, the individual state) that grants individuals the right to practice. Licensing requirements vary widely from state to state, and they are changing rapidly. Thirty-eight states license Oriental medicine practitioners and acupuncturists. Most of them use the NCCAOM exam as their standard. Licensing is usually achieved by meeting educational and exam requirements.

The nationwide trend in acupuncture and Oriental medicine is toward more education and stricter certification and licensing requirements. The profession is developing the Doctor of Oriental Medicine designation, which should be available in the near future. The national professional organizations can provide the most up-to-date information about certification and licensing issues.

If your career is in Oriental bodywork, you must be aware that the individual states regulate Oriental bodywork practitioners as they do general massage therapists. Twenty-five states and the District of Columbia license massage therapists. They generally require completion of a 500-hour program and the National Certification Exam for Therapeutic Massage and Bodywork. The American Massage Therapy Association can give you information regarding the laws of your state. If your state does not have licensing requirements, check with your county or municipality for regulations governing massage therapy.

The American Oriental Bodywork Therapy Association offers two certifications in Oriental bodywork to those who meet their membership requirements. Membership qualifications vary according to the type and level of membership sought. The AOBTA designates certified practitioners (minimum of 500 hours training) and associates (minimum of 150 hours training). The Oriental bodywork training hours are in addition to the hours required for a general massage license.

Other Requirements

Oriental medicine practitioners work with people who may be ill or in pain. To be a good health care practitioner, you need to have compassion and understanding for your clients. You need a strong desire to help people improve their lives. Good listening skills and a reassuring manner are important. Strong intuition, careful observation, and good problem-solving skills are also valuable.

Oriental medicine is a science of understanding energetics in the body, and it is a healing art. Whether you pursue a career as an Oriental bodywork therapist or as an acupuncturist, you need to be successful at understanding and learning this approach to health care. Oriental medicine practitioners who specialize in acupuncture need sensitive hands and keen vision. Those who specialize in Oriental bodywork need strong hands and physical stamina.

Exploring

Study Oriental history, thought, and philosophy to help you learn to understand Oriental medicine's approach to healing. Watch videos and read about or take courses in t'ai qi, kung fu, or other forms of qigong. Begin to experience these ancient methods for achieving control of the mind and body that will be part of your studies in Oriental medicine. Health food stores have books on acupuncture, Chinese herbology, and perhaps on Oriental bodywork. You can learn about other alternative or complementary health modalities. Visit Chinese herb shops.

Talk with people who have experienced acupuncture, Chinese herbal therapy, or Oriental bodywork therapy. Find out what it was like and how they felt about it. Make an appointment for a health consultation with an Oriental medicine practitioner. Find out if this approach to health care works for you, and if you would like to use it to help others.

Visit colleges of Oriental medicine or massage schools. Sit in on classes. Talk to the students. Ask what they like and what they don't like about the schools. Investigate the national and state professional associations. Many of them have excellent Web sites. Some have student memberships. Attend meetings and get to know the people and the issues in the field. Network with experienced acupuncturists or Oriental bodyworkers. Try to find a mentor.

Employers

Most Oriental medicine practitioners who specialize in acupuncture, Chinese herbology, or other modalities of Oriental medicine operate private practices. Some form or join partnerships with other Oriental medicine practitioners or with practitioners of other alternative health care modalities. Professionals at clinics in other areas of health care, such as chiropractors, osteopaths, and MDs, increasingly include Oriental medicine practitioners.

As Oriental medicine and acupuncture become more accepted, there are growing opportunities for practitioners in hospitals and university medical schools. A few are engaged in medical research. They conduct studies on the effectiveness of Oriental medicine in treating various health conditions. There is a growing emphasis on research in acupuncture, and this area is likely to employ more people in the future. A few Oriental medicine practitioners work for government agencies, such as the National Institutes of Health.

Oriental bodywork therapists practice in clinics with acupuncturists, other Oriental medicine practitioners, or other alternative health practitioners. They also work in many of the locations where conventional massage therapists practice: conventional doctors' offices, gyms, hotels, spas, cruise ships, fitness centers, nursing homes, and hospitals. Some establish private practices or run their own clinics. A few teach Oriental bodywork in massage schools or in programs that specialize in Oriental bodywork.

Starting Out

When you start out as an Oriental medicine practitioner—whether as an Oriental bodywork therapist or as an acupuncturist—one of the most important considerations is having the proper certification and licensing for your geographical area. This is essential because the requirements for the professions, for each state, and for the nation are changing rapidly.

The placement office of your school may be able to help you find job opportunities. When starting out, acupuncturists sometimes find jobs in clinics with alternative health care practitioners or chiropractors or in wellness centers. This gives them a chance to start practicing in a setting where they can work with and learn from others. Some begin working with more experienced practitioners and then later go into private practice. Oriental medicine practitioners frequently work in private practice. When starting new practices, they often have full-time jobs and begin their practices part time.

Oriental bodywork therapists may also find work in clinics with chiropractors or other complementary health care practitioners. In addition, they might find job opportunities in local health clubs, spas, nursing homes, hospitals, or wellness centers. Networking with professionals in local and national organizations is always a good way to learn about job opportunities. Join the organizations that interest you, attend meetings, and get to know people in the field.

Advancement

Oriental medicine practitioners who specialize in acupuncture or Chinese herbology advance in their careers by establishing their own practices, by building large bases of patients, and by starting their own clinics. Because they receive referrals from physicians and other alternative health care practitioners, relationships with other members of the medical community are very helpful in building a patient base.

Very experienced acupuncturists may teach at a school of Oriental medicine. After much experience, an individual may achieve a supervisory or directorship position in a school. The growing acceptance of acupuncture and Oriental medicine by the American public and the medical community will lead to an increasing need for research in university medical hospitals or government agencies.

For Oriental medicine practitioners who specialize in Oriental bodywork, advancement can come in the form of promotions within the facility where they work—resort, health club, or health care facilities. They can take more advanced courses and pursue an upper-level BA specialty in Oriental bodywork. They, too, can advance by becoming teachers or starting their own businesses.

Earnings

Starting pay for a private practitioner specializing in acupuncture and Oriental medicine may be $13,000 to $20,000 until the practice expands. As with other forms of self-employment, income is directly related to the number of hours you work and the rate you can charge. Rates increase with experience. Clinics might offer $15,000 to $20,000 to start. Average income for full-time acupuncturists is $35,000 to $50,000. Very experienced Oriental medicine practitioners with well-established practices can net $200,000 or more.

Oriental bodywork therapists' earnings depend upon the setting in which they work. Those who work in the same locations where conventional massage therapists are employed may have similar incomes. Massage therapists earnings range from $10,700 for entry level to $40,000 for mid-level and up to $72,800 for very experienced. Oriental bodywork therapists who are self-employed can charge around $40 per hour when starting out. Mid-level therapists can charge $65 and very experienced therapists may earn as much as $125 per hour. Most Oriental bodywork sessions last a full hour, so therapists' incomes are limited by the number of sessions they schedule.

Work Environment

Oriental bodywork therapists work in a variety of settings, and the work environment can vary greatly. In most locations, they work indoors in clean, comfortable surroundings. Solo practitioners may set up their own offices or travel to their clients' homes or places of business. If they have to travel, they frequently charge a travel fee. They have flexible schedules and can set their own hours. Being self-employed, they must provide their own benefits.

Oriental bodywork therapists who work in doctors' offices, in hospitals, on cruise ships, in spas, or for other employers usually work more regular hours, depending upon their employers' demands. They may receive benefits. Weekend and evening hours may be required to meet the needs of clients.

Oriental medicine practitioners who specialize in acupuncture usually work indoors in clean, quiet, comfortable offices. Since most are in private practice, they define their own surroundings. Private practitioners set their own hours, but many work some evenings or weekends to accommodate their patients' schedules. They usually work without supervision and must have a lot of self-discipline. Like other self-employed individuals, acupuncturists must provide their own insurance, vacation, and retirement benefits.

For acupuncturists who work in clinics, hospitals, universities, and research settings, the surroundings vary. They may work in large hospitals or small colleges. However, wherever they work, health care practitioners need clean, quiet offices. In these larger settings, practitioners need to be good team players. They may also need to be able to work well under supervision. Those who are employed in these organizations usually receive salaries and benefits. They may have to follow hours set by the employer.

Outlook

All aspects of Oriental medicine are growing rapidly due to increasing public awareness and acceptance. Interest from the mainstream medical community, recent advances in research, and favorable changes in government policy are strong indicators that the field will continue to expand. As insurance, health maintenance organization (HMO), and other third-party reimbursements increase, Oriental medicine is expected to grow even more rapidly. In 1997, the World Health Organization (the medical branch of the United Nations) estimated that there were over 10,000 acupuncture specialists in the United States. The number of certified and licensed acupuncturists and Oriental medicine practitioners is expected to increase as additional states establish legal guidelines.

The number of people who seek Oriental medicine practitioners of acupuncture for their health care needs is growing annually. Oriental medicine is used to relieve a wide range of common ailments, including asthma, high blood pressure, headache, and back pain. Many Americans turn to Oriental medicine practitioners for internal medicine, oncology, obstetrics/gynecology, pediatrics, urology, geriatrics, sports medicine, immunology, infectious diseases, and psychiatric disorders. The demand for Oriental medicine practitioners specializing in acupuncture is growing much faster than the average for all occupations.

As an important part of Oriental medicine, Oriental bodywork therapy also has a bright future. As more alternative health care practitioners enter practice in response to public demand, positions for Oriental bodywork therapy will increase. Alternative health care practitioners, such as chiropractors and holistic physicians, are good sources of employment and referrals for Oriental bodywork therapists.

The national emphasis on wellness and natural health care promises to keep the demand for Oriental bodywork therapists and other Oriental medicine practitioners increasing faster than the average in the first decade of the 21st century.

For More Information

For general information, a list of schools offering Oriental medicine programs, and a Web site with good links, contact:

American Association of Oriental Medicine
433 Front Street
Catasauqua, PA 18032
Tel: 610-266-1433
Web: http://www.aaom.org

For information regarding state regulations for massage therapists and general information on therapeutic massage, contact:

American Massage Therapy Association
820 Davis Street, Suite 100
Evanston, IL 60201-4444
Tel: 847-864-0123
Web: http://www.amtamassage.org/

To learn more about Oriental bodywork, national and regional workshops, and a practitioner referral service contact:

American Oriental Bodywork Therapy Association
Laurel Oak Corporate Center, Suite 408
1010 Haddonfield-Berlin Road
Voorhees, NJ 08043
Tel: 609-782-1616
Web: http://www.healthworld.com/associations/pa/bodywork/about1.htm

For information for potential students, general information about Oriental medicine, and comprehensive information about national organizations, changes in legislation, and state standards, contact:

National Acupuncture and Oriental Medicine Alliance
14637 Starr Road, SE
Olalla, WA 98359
Tel: 253-851-6896
Web: http://www.acuall.org

To learn more about qigong and to connect with the qigong community in the United States through a discussion forum, contact:

National Qigong Association
PO Box 20218
Boulder Springs, CO 80308
Tel: 888-218-7788
Web: http://www.nqa.org

Osteopaths

Biology Psychology	School Subjects
Helping/teaching Technical/scientific	Personal Skills
Primarily indoors Primarily one location	Work Environment
Medical degree	Minimum Education Level
$35,000 to $166,000 to $250,000+	Salary Range
Required by all states	Certification or Licensing
Much faster than the average	Outlook

Overview

Osteopaths practice a medical discipline that uses refined and sophisticated manipulative therapy based on the late 19th century teachings of American Dr. Andrew Taylor Still. It embraces the idea of "whole person" medicine and looks upon the system of muscles, bones, and joints—particularly the spine—as reflecting the body's diseases and as being partially responsible for initiating disease processes. Osteopaths are medical doctors with additional specialized training in this unique approach. They practice in a wide range of fields, from environmental medicine, geriatrics, and nutrition to sports medicine and neurology, among others.

History

Osteopathy has its roots in the hardships and challenges of 19th-century America. Its developer, Dr. Andrew Taylor Still, was born in 1828 in Virginia, the son of a Methodist minister and physician. There were few medical schools in the United States, so Still received his early medical training largely from his father. As the Civil War began, he attended the College of Physicians and Surgeons in Kansas City, but he enlisted in the army before completing the course.

In 1864, an epidemic of meningitis struck the Missouri frontier. Thousands died, including Still's three children. His inability to help them underscored his growing dissatisfaction with traditional medical approaches. After much careful study of anatomy, physiology, and the general nature of health, he became convinced that cultivating a deep understanding of the structure-function relationship between the parts of the body was the only path to a true understanding of disease. Eventually, Still came to believe in three basic principles that would form the core of his osteopathic approach to the practice of medicine. First, he saw the body as capable of self-healing, producing its own healing substances. Second, he felt health was dependent upon the structural integrity of the body. And, finally, because of these beliefs, he considered distorted structure a fundamental cause of disease.

A system of physical manipulation was an integral component of Still's new practice. He began to compare manipulative therapy with other methods then used by doctors, such as drugs and surgery. Often, he found the use of manipulative methods made drugs and operations unnecessary. Instead, he focused on the musculoskeletal system—the muscles, bones, nerves, and ligaments. Recognizing that structural misalignments often occurred in these areas, he emphasized the system's importance as a major potential factor in disease, ripe for the application of his new manipulative techniques.

Still founded the first college of osteopathy in Kirksville, Missouri, in 1892, basing it upon the fundamental principles of his osteopathic concept. Fewer than 20 men and women graduated from this first osteopathic college in 1894. Today, there are 18 osteopathic schools in the United States. Some are part of major university campuses, and combined, they accept roughly 2,500 new osteopathic students annually.

Andrew Still died in 1917, leaving behind a legacy of enormous importance to the history of medicine. Medicine as we know it was in its infancy in his day, and theories, tools, and techniques we take for granted now— such as the concept of germs, the use of antiseptics, and the diagnostic possibilities presented by radiology—were just beginning. In this challenging environment, Still worked out a practical system of structural therapeutics that has withstood the pressure of later discoveries.

Although practitioners of alternative methods of healing in the United States were—and sometimes still are—seen as a threat by the medical profession, osteopathy has increased in popularity. As the field grew, some students wished to use drugs as well as osteopathic techniques in treating patients. John Martin Littlejohn, for example—a Scotsman who studied with Still—widened the focus of osteopathy by concentrating not only on anatomy, but stressing physiological aspects as well. Unlike Still, Littlejohn wanted osteopaths to learn all about modern medicine, along with osteopathic principles and practices. Later, Littlejohn returned to Britain, where he founded the British School of Osteopathy. Even so, the training of osteopaths in the United States was, in fact, eventually to merge with the training of orthodox medical physicians.

The Job

Osteopathy and orthodox medicine both use the scientific knowledge of anatomy and physiology, as well as clinical methods of investigation. In this respect, they have a similar language. The greatest differences, however, lie in the way patients are evaluated and in the approach to treatment. As a general rule, the orthodox medical approach focuses on the end result of the problem: the illness. Treatments seek to repair the imbalance presented by the illness through the prescription of drugs or by surgery. In contrast, osteopaths focus on tracing the changes in a patient's ability to function that have occurred over a period of time. This is done to understand the chain of events that have altered the relationship between structure and function, resulting in the patient's present complaint. The primary aim of treatment is to remove the obstacles within a patient's body that are preventing the natural self-healing process from occurring. It's a subtle difference, but important.

Like most physicians, as an osteopath, you'll probably spend much of your day seeing patients in a clinic or hospital setting. Your specialty, of course, may take you to other venues—nursing homes or sports arenas, for instance.

Your first task in evaluating a new patient is trying to understand the cause of the problem that the patient presents. It may sound simple, but it can be very complex. Diagnosis is a fluid art and treatment programs are reviewed with each patient visit, changing as the patient begins to respond. To arrive at an appropriate diagnosis, the history you take as an osteopath will likely be greatly detailed—remember, the osteopath needs to consider the whole body. Since structure and function are interdependent, and all the parts of the body connect with each other, you may find yourself asking questions that appear to have little relevance to the problem at hand. It is precisely that concern for seemingly irrelevant details, coupled with manipulative therapy, which distinguishes the osteopath (or D.O.) from the allopath (or conventional M.D.)

One technique that assists in the correct evaluation of patient problems is palpation, a manual means of diagnosis and determination, whereby sensory information is received through the fingers and hands. Along with careful listening and observation, palpation will help you assess healthy tissue and identify structural problems or painful areas in your patient's body.

The osteopath differs from a traditional M.D. or allopathic physician in one other major aspect—that is, with respect to treatment options. For the D.O., treatment centers around what are called osteopathic lesions. Osteopathic lesions are functional disturbances in the body, involving muscles, joints, and other body systems. They are not lesions as M.D.s refer to them—incursions, cuts, or other tissue damage—but are created by mechanical and physiological reactions in the body to various types of trauma. In osteopathy, open, unhindered, and balanced movement is the most important factor in health. The lack of it plays a major role in the onset of disease and illness. Thus, the many varied techniques employed by osteopaths are concerned primarily with re-establishing normal mobility and removing or reducing the underlying lesions.

As an osteopath, the techniques available to you to address osteopathic lesions are nearly limitless. Treatment techniques can be flexible in their application; because your guide for choice is the patient's body, each application of a particular technique, however, will be unique. Similar lesions in different patients will have different origins and will have been caused by different sorts of forces or events. Your thorough evaluation of the patient will help guide you in discerning what sorts of techniques will be most helpful.

Requirements

High School

Students who plan a career as a physician—either as a D.O. or an M.D.—should take a college preparatory program in high school. You'll need a strong foundation in the sciences, especially biology, chemistry, and physics. In addition, take English, history, foreign languages, and all the math you can. Psychology is a helpful course in preparing you to work well with a wide variety of people coming to you for treatment. Strive to become as well-rounded an individual as possible.

Postsecondary Training

For persons with bachelor's degrees, the American Association of Colleges of Osteopathic Medicine offers prospective medical students a centralized application service for the 19 accredited osteopathic medical schools. Students file one application along with a single set of transcripts and MCAT (Medical College Admission Test) scores. The service will verify and distribute your application to those colleges you designate. You should be aware that admission to an osteopathic medical school, like all medical schools, is quite competitive. Over 9,500 applicants submitted a total of more than 55,000 applications in 1997. Only a combined total of 2,500 seats were available to first-year students.

Once you're in, the academic program leading to the Doctor of Osteopathy degree involves four years of study, followed by a one-year rotating internship in areas such as internal medicine, obstetrics/gynecology, and surgery. If you're interested in a specific specialty, an additional two to six years of residency training is required.

The curriculum in colleges of osteopathic medicine supports Dr. Still's osteopathic philosophy, with an emphasis on preventive, family, and community medicine. Clinical instruction stresses examining all patient characteristics (including behavioral and environmental), and how various body systems interrelate. Close attention is given to the ways in which the musculoskeletal and nervous systems influence the functioning of the entire body. An increasing emphasis on biomedical research in several of the colleges has expanded opportunities for students wishing to pursue research careers.

Certification or Licensing

At an early point in the residency period, all physicians, both M.D.s and D.O.s, must pass a state medical board examination in order to obtain a license and enter practice. Each state sets its own requirements and issues its own licenses, although some states will accept licenses from other states.

Many osteopathic physicians belong to the American Osteopathic Association (AOA). To retain membership, physicians must complete 150 hours of continuing education every three years. Continuing education can be acquired in a variety of ways, including attending professional conferences, completing education programs sponsored by the AOA, osteopathic medical teaching, and publishing articles in professional journals.

The AOA offers board certification. Certification has many requirements, including passing a comprehensive written exam as a well as a practical test in which you must demonstrate osteopathic manipulative techniques. The AOA offers specialty certification in more than 100 specialty areas. Some osteopathic physicians are certified by both the AOA and the American Medical Association (AMA).

Other Requirements

There are a few other things to keep in mind if you're considering a career in osteopathy. For instance, the practice of osteopathy usually involves a lot of personal interaction, and a lot of touching, which can make some patients— and some prospective doctors—feel uncomfortable. Osteopathic physicians need excellent communication skills to tell patients what to expect and what is happening at any one moment. Good communication skills are also necessary to do the best job informing your patients about the right kind of treatment. If patients don't understand what you're telling them, they may not pursue the treatment. You need to learn to work well with others and to be a perceptive listener.

Since a large number of osteopaths go into private practice, business and management skills are useful. In addition, good manual dexterity is important to use manipulative techniques for the patient's optimum benefit. Finally, and most importantly, you must have a real commitment to caring for people in this way. A lesser goal may not be enough to help see you through the sometimes difficult and always long days of training.

Exploring

Consider visiting an osteopathic medical college. Tours are often available and can give you extra insight into necessary training and the ways in which life at an osteopathic medical school differs from a "regular" one. If you don't live close enough to an osteopathic college to visit, write for more information.

Check into after-school or summer jobs at your local hospital or medical center. Any job that exposes you to the care of patients is a good one, even jobs you might not think of at first, or ones that aren't exactly medical, such as working with the janitorial service. Contact the American Osteopathic Association and ask for a list of osteopaths in your area. Talk to as many people as you can and don't be afraid to ask questions.

Employers

Osteopaths can be found in virtually all medical specialties. They use the most modern scientific methods to understand and treat their patients' problems, and this means they often are hired by a wide variety of institutions. Many—more than one-third—go into private practice after completing their training. They also work in hospitals, clinics, nursing homes, and other health care settings. Anywhere you can find an M.D., you probably also can find a D.O.

Starting Out

For a newly graduated physician, the first step beyond medical school and internship is additional schooling. Depending upon the specialty in which you're interested, you can plan on completing a residency program of two to six years' duration. Gaining admission to the program you want may be a challenge. One of the difficulties facing the profession today is that its schools produce more students than there are available spaces for residents at osteopathic hospitals. Graduates of osteopathic hospitals must increasingly find residencies in traditional medical facilities—where some osteopaths feel that it's more difficult to adhere to the unique philosophy that is central to their training. As awareness of and interest in osteopathy continue to grow, this situation may change. After residency, you can choose to go into private practice or explore positions with a variety of health care employers.

Advancement

Advancement in the medical professions is dependent on the specific field you're in. Osteopaths in private practice will follow a different career path than those working in a purely clinical setting, who live still a different life than osteopaths who choose a research-oriented career at an academic medical center. As noted earlier, a large percentage of osteopaths go into private or small-group practice. Advancement in private practice is largely what you make of it. As your practice grows, you'll earn the satisfaction of knowing patients in your community are well cared for. You'll set your career goals yourself.

In contrast, osteopaths in employee positions are more limited by the type of job they've taken. Osteopaths in an academic setting, like any physician-teacher, face the challenge of obtaining tenure and advance on a track from instructor to assistant professor to associate professor to professor. Becoming tenured is an arduous process, involving a combination of patient care, research and publication, and administrative responsibilities. If you love the academic environment, however, and also want to be a practicing physician, you may find your niche in academia.

Earnings

Osteopaths earn incomes comparable to their M.D. counterparts, and the potentially high income of an established physician can be an enticing perk of becoming an osteopath. Median net income (after expenses but before taxes) in 1996 was $166,000 for all M.D.s in clinical practice. Some make less, many make more. There are a number of other factors you might want to keep in mind, however, as described in a recent survey of the American Medical Association. Counting postgraduate education, most physicians are in their early thirties before starting to practice. Residency pay is low, yet residents worked an average of 80 to 100 hours per week. Most physicians incur high educational debt by the time they begin to practice. Eighty-two percent of 1996 graduates reported some level of debt, with the average amounting to $75,103.

Benefits for osteopathic physicians vary, depending on whether they work in private practice or for an employer. In general, it depends, too, on how you define benefits. The AMA survey indicates that median net income for self-employed physicians is approximately 40 percent higher than that of employee physicians. Many factors contribute to the difference. Self-employed physicians tend to be older, have more years of experience, work more hours, and are more likely to be board certified, all of which are associated with higher earnings. On the other hand, 75 percent of employee physicians receive noncash benefits in addition to their reported income, whereas some self-employed physicians do not. These benefits represent approximately 5 percent of income for employees.

Work Environment

As with the benefits you earn, the environment in which you work can vary as an osteopath. During your training, you will be highly supervised; eventually you will be deemed to have garnered the knowledge necessary to work on your own. In both private practice and employer-based situations, you will sometimes work alone (e.g., directly with your patient) and sometimes be part of a team. Osteopathy, like all medical professions, is a field of contrasts, requiring both collaboration and personal insight. If you enjoy the idea of becoming a physician, a wide array of work environments will be open to you as an osteopath. What's the primary obstacle to be aware of going in? It's no surprise: some extraordinarily long hours, particularly during training.

Outlook

The records of the American Association of Colleges of Osteopathic Medicine show the number of osteopathic graduates has increased 50 percent in the last decade, making osteopathic medicine one of the fastest-growing health professions in the country. To meet the growing demand, more than a dozen new osteopathic medical colleges have opened their doors since the mid-1970s. Together, all 19 institutions currently enroll more than 8,000 students annually, of whom nearly 35 percent are women.

Although osteopathic medicine is not strictly an "alternative" approach, the field is benefiting from the current interest in these kinds of therapies. Excellent job opportunities will continue to become available for skilled osteopathic physicians. In addition to specialized practices in areas such as family medicine, increasing interest in biomedical research at the osteopathic colleges also is expanding opportunities for candidates interested in careers in medical research.

For More Information

The AACOM offers a wide array of resources to high school and college students interested in a career in osteopathy. In addition to its centralized application service, the association publishes a college information booklet and a financial aid guide. A good deal of general information is accessible through the association's Web site, so it's a good place to start your search.

American Association of Colleges of Osteopathic Medicine
5550 Friendship Boulevard, Suite 310
Chevy Chase, MD 20815
Tel: 301-968-4100
Web: http:\\www.aacom.org

The AOA is a clearinghouse for general information about osteopathy and the ways it can help to keep you healthy. Its Web site offers many short booklets on family health topics as well as osteopathic medicine.

American Osteopathic Association
Department of Communications
142 East Ontario Street
Chicago, IL 60611
Tel: 312-202-8000 or 800-621-1773
Web: http:\\www.am-osteo-assn.org

Reflexologists

	School Subjects
Biology Health Psychology	

	Personal Skills
Communication/ideas Helping/teaching	

	Work Environment
Primarily indoors Primarily one location	

	Minimum Education Level
High school diploma	

	Salary Range
$7,000 to $35,000 to $100,000+	

	Certification or Licensing
Recommended	

	Outlook
Much faster than the average	

Overview

Reflexologists base their work on the theory that "reflexes," specific points on the hands and feet, correspond to specific points on other parts of the body. They apply pressure to the feet or hands of their clients in order to affect the areas of the body that correspond to the areas that they are manipulating. Reflexologists believe that their work promotes overall good health, helps clients relax, and speeds the healing process.

History

Reflexology—or something similar to it—was practiced thousands of years ago. More than 2,000 years before the common era, the Chinese learned that foot massage was a useful adjunct to the practice of acupuncture. Many modern practitioners of reflexology believe that reflexology utilizes the principles on which acupuncture and traditional Chinese medicine (TCM) are based. A 4,000-year-old fresco that appears in the tomb of Ankhmahor, physician to a pharaoh, in the Egyptian city of Saqqara depicts the practice of foot massage. In North America, the Cherokee people have emphasized the importance of the feet in health, partly because it is through the feet that human beings connect with the earth. Zone theory, which provides the theoretical basis for reflexology, existed in Europe as early as the 1500s.

Although reflexology is an ancient practice, its modern form originated in the early 20th century. William Fitzgerald, a Connecticut-based physician who was an ear, nose, and throat specialist, revived the practice of reflexology in the West in 1913, when he found that applying pressure to a patient's hands or feet just before surgery decreased the level of pain experienced by the patient. In 1917, Fitzgerald wrote *Zone Therapy, or Relieving Pain at Home,* which described his work. Fitzgerald believed that "bioelectrical energy" flows from points in the feet or hands to specific points elsewhere in the body, and he thought that applying tourniquets and various instruments to the feet or hands enhanced the flow of energy. He set out to map the flow of that energy, and in the process he set up correspondences between areas on the feet or hands and areas throughout the body.

The next important figure in modern reflexology, Eunice Ingham, was a physiotherapist who had worked with Joseph Shelby Riley, a follower of William Fitzgerald. Riley had decided against using instruments to manipulate the feet and hands, opting to use his hands instead. Ingham practiced and taught extensively, mapped the correspondences between the reflexes and the parts of the body, and wrote books chronicling her work with her patients, which helped to promote the field of reflexology. She went on to found the organization now known as the International Institute of Reflexology (IIR), which continues to promote the Original Ingham Method of Reflexology. Ultimately, Ingham became known as the mother of modern reflexology. Her students have played major roles in spreading reflexology throughout the world.

The Job

Reflexologists believe that the standing human body is divided vertically into ten zones, five zones on each side of the imaginary vertical line that divides the body in two. On both sides, the zone closest to the middle is zone one, while the zone farthest from the middle is zone five. These zones also appear on the hands and feet. Reflexologists believe that by massaging a spot in a zone on the foot, they can stimulate a particular area in the corresponding zone of the body. By massaging the reflex in the middle of the big toe, for example, a reflexologist attempts to affect the pituitary gland, which is the corresponding body part.

Reflexologists also believe that their ministrations help their clients in two other ways. First, they believe that their treatments reduce the amount of lactic acid in the feet. Lactic acid is a natural waste product of the metabolic process, and its presence in large quantities is unhealthful. Second, they believe that their treatments break up calcium crystals that have built up in the nerve endings of the feet. It is their theory that the presence of these crystals inhibits the flow of energy, which is increased when the crystals are removed. Reflexologists also emphasize that their techniques improve circulation and promote relaxation.

It is worth noting that modern science has not validated the theoretical basis of reflexology, which is even less well accepted in the scientific world than are some other alternative therapies. Yet it is also worth noting that some therapies whose underlying theories have not been validated by science have been shown to be effective. Relatively few scientific studies of reflexology have been completed, but much research is underway at present, and it is likely that reflexology will be better understood in the near future.

An initial visit to a reflexologist generally begins with the practitioner asking the client questions about his or her overall health, medical problems, and the reason for the visit. The reflexologist makes the client comfortable and begins the examination and treatment.

Although most reflexologists, such as the followers of Eunice Ingham, work on their clients' feet or hands with their hands, some prefer to use instruments. In either case, the reflexologist works on the feet and looks for sore spots, which are thought to indicate illness or other problems in the corresponding part of the body. On occasion, the problem will not be manifested in the corresponding organ or part of the body, but will instead be manifested elsewhere within the zone. Usually, the reflexologist will spend more time on the sore spots than on other parts of the foot. On the basis of information provided by the client and information obtained by the reflexologist during the examination, the reflexologist will recommend a course of treatment that is appropriate for the client's physical condition. In some cases, such as those of extreme illness, the reflexologist may ask the client to check with his or her physician to determine whether the treatment may be in conflict with the physician's course of treatment. Most reflexologists will not treat a client who has a fever. In addition, because reflexology treatments tend to enhance circulation, it is sometimes necessary for a client who is taking medication to decrease the dosage, on the advice of a doctor, to compensate for the increased circulation and the resulting increased effectiveness of the medication.

One of the most important aspects of the reflexologist's skill is knowing exactly how much pressure to apply to a person's feet. The pressure required for a large, healthy adult, for example, would be too much for a young child or a baby. Different foot shapes and weights may also require different levels of pressure. The practitioner must also know how long to work on the foot, since the benefits of the treatment may be offset if the treatment lasts too long. In her book *Reflexology Today*, Doreen E. Bayly, one of Eunice Ingham's students, recalled that Ingham once told her: "If you work on the reflex too long, you are undoing the good you have done." Ingham recommended 30-minute sessions, but most modern reflexologists conduct 45-minute or 60-minute sessions unless the client's condition dictates otherwise.

Most reflexologists work primarily on feet, but some work on the hands or even the ears. If a foot has been injured or amputated, it is acceptable to work on the hands. For the most part, reflexologists work on the feet because the feet are so sensitive. In addition, feet that are encased in shoes during most of the day typically require more attention than hands do. Furthermore, the feet, because of their size, are easier to manipulate. It is somewhat more difficult to find the reflexes on the hands.

Requirements

High School

Because the practice of reflexology involves utilizing the correspondences between reflexes and the various parts of the body, a student who has some knowledge of medicine and anatomy will be ahead of the game. A student who wishes to become a reflexologist would do well to study biology, chemistry, and health—anything that relates to the medical sciences. Since reflexologists must make their clients comfortable and gain their trust, some study of psychology may be useful. An interested high school student would also do well to investigate areas of bodywork and alternative medicine that are not taught in school. A student who has some knowledge of or practical skill in some area of massage (shiatsu, Swedish massage, and so forth) will have a head start, especially since some states require reflexologists to be licensed massage therapists.

Postsecondary Training

The single most important part of a reflexologist's training is the completion of a rigorous course of study and practice, such as that provided by the International Institute of Reflexology. Many courses are available, and they range from one-day sessions designed to train people to work on themselves or their partners to comprehensive courses that require a commitment of nine months or longer on the part of the student. Naturally, a student who wishes to practice professionally should select a comprehensive course. Correspondence courses are available, but any reputable correspondence course will require that the student complete a required number of hours of supervised, hands-on work. Some aspects of the technique must be demonstrated, not simply read, especially concerning the amount of pressure that the reflexologist should apply to different kinds of feet. Many reflexologists offer services other than reflexology, and the student may wish to be trained in aromatherapy or in various kinds of bodywork. Such training may also increase the likelihood that the practitioner, especially at the beginning of his or her career, will make a decent living.

Certification or Licensing

In some states, such as North Dakota, a reflexologist who has completed a course given by a reputable school of reflexology can be licensed specifically as a reflexologist. In most states, however, reflexologists are subject to the laws that govern massage therapists. That often means that a reflexologist must complete a state-certified course in massage before being licensed to practice reflexology. In many cases, reflexologists are subject to laws that are designed to regulate "massage parlors" that are fronts for prostitution. In some places, these laws require that practitioners be subjected to disease testing and walk-in inspections by police. It is common for those who are medical doctors or licensed cosmetologists to be exempt from massage-licensing regulations. Because there is such wide variation in the law, anyone who wishes to practice reflexology should carefully study state and local regulations before setting up shop.

Reflexologists-to-be should enroll in a course that requires a substantial number of hours of training and certifies the student upon graduation. Those who are at least 18 years old, have a high school diploma or its equivalent, have completed a course that requires at least 110 hours of training, and have at least 90 documented postgraduate reflexology sessions under their belts can apply to be tested by the American Reflexology Certification Board (ARCB), which was created in 1991. The organization is designed to promote reflexology by recognizing competent practitioners. Testing is purely voluntary, but a high score from the ARCB is certainly a good sign that a practitioner is competent.

Other Requirements

Reflexologists work closely with their clients, so it is essential that they be friendly, open, and sensitive to the feelings of others. They must be able to gain their clients' trust, make them comfortable and relaxed, and communicate well enough with them to gather the information that they need in order to treat them effectively. It is highly unlikely that an uncommunicative person who is uncomfortable with people will be able to build a reflexology practice. A reflexologist who practices in a state that has licensing regulations that require training in a field such as massage must also be able to complete that training. In addition, a reflexologist must be comfortable making decisions and working alone. Most reflexologists have their own practices, and anyone who sets up shop will need to deal with the basic tasks and problems that all business owners face: advertising, accounting, taxes, legal requirements, and so forth.

Exploring

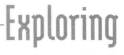

The best way to learn about the field of reflexology is to speak with reflexologists. Call practitioners and ask to interview them. Find reflexologists in your area if you can, but do not hesitate to contact people in other areas. There is no substitute for learning from those who actually do the work. Although most reflexologists run one-person practices, it may be possible to find clerical work of some kind with a successful practitioner in your area, especially if you live in a large city.

You should also do as much reading as you can on the subject. Many books are currently available, and many more will be available in the near future, since the field is growing rapidly. Look for information on reflexology in magazines that deal with alternative medicine and bodywork. Learn as much as you can about alternative therapies. You may find that you wish to practice a number of techniques in addition to reflexology.

Employers

For the most part, reflexologists work for themselves, although they may work at businesses that include reflexology as one of a number of services that they provide. It is probably wise to assume that you are going to run your own business, even if you do end up working for another organization. In most cases, organizations that use reflexologists bring them in as independent contractors rather than employees.

Starting Out

You should begin by taking the best, most comprehensive course of study you can find from a school that will certify you as a practitioner. After that, if you have not found an organization that you can work for, you should begin to practice on your own. You may rent an office or set up shop at home in order to save money. You may begin by working part-time, so that you can earn money by other means while you are getting your business underway. Be sure to investigate the state and local laws that may affect you.

A reflexologist who runs his or her own business needs to be well versed in basic business skills. You may want to take courses in business or seek advice from the local office of the Small Business Administration. Seek advice from people you know who run their own businesses. Your financial survival will depend on your business skills, so be sure that you know what you are doing.

Advancement

Because most reflexologists work for themselves, advancement in the field is directly related to the quality of treatment they provide and their business skills. The best way to get ahead as a reflexologist is to prove to the members of your community that you are skilled, honest, professional, and effective. Only when there is a strong demand for your services can you expect to thrive financially. When you have attained a high level of skill and your clients are urging their friends to take their business to you, financial success is probable.

Earnings

There are no reliable figures to indicate what reflexologists earn per year. In most cases, however, reflexologists charge between $30 and $60 per hour. Some practitioners may charge as little as $15 per hour, while a small number of well-respected reflexologists in large cities may earn $100 or even substantially more per hour. Many reflexologists do not work 40 hours per week doing reflexology exclusively. It is likely that most reflexologists earn between $7,000 and $35,000 per year, while some may earn more than $100,000 per year. Typically, it takes quite some time for new practitioners to build up a practice, so many of them rely on other sources of income in the beginning. Many reflexologists offer other holistic treatments and therapies, which means that they do not rely on reflexology to provide all their income.

Work Environment

Reflexologists almost always work in their homes or in their own offices. Although some reflexologists may have office help, most work alone. For this reason, practitioners must be independent enough to work effectively on schedules of their own devising. Because they must make their clients comfortable in order to provide effective treatment, they generally try to make their workplaces as pleasant and relaxing as possible. Many practitioners play soothing music while they work. Some—especially those who practice aromatherapy as well as reflexology—use scents to create an attractive atmosphere.

Outlook

Although no official government analysis of the future of reflexology has yet been conducted, it seems safe to say that the field is expanding much more rapidly than the average for all fields. Although science still views it with skepticism, reflexology has become relatively popular in a short period of time. It has certainly benefited from the popular acceptance of alternative medicine and therapies in recent years, particularly because it is a holistic practice that aims to treat the whole person rather than the symptoms of disease or discomfort. Because reflexology treatments entail little risk to the client in most cases, they provide a safe and convenient way to improve health.

For More Information

The IIR promotes the Original Ingham Method of Reflexology, providing seminars worldwide as well as a thorough certification program. The Institute also sells books and charts.

The International Institute of Reflexology
PO Box 12642
St. Petersburg, FL 33733-2642
Tel: 727-343-4811
Web: http://ourworld.compuserve.com/homepages/Mike Levick/

The ARCB was created in order to promote reflexology by recognizing competent practitioners. It provides voluntary testing for working reflexologists and maintains lists of certified practitioners.

American Reflexology Certification Board
PO Box 620607
Littleton, CO 80162
Tel: 303-933-6921

Laura Norman's organization provides training and certification in reflexology. It also sells books, reflexology products, and aromatherapy supplies.

Laura Norman and Associates
41 Park Avenue, Suite 8A
New York, NY 10016
Tel: 212-532-4404
Web: http://lauranormanrefloxology.com

Index